THE ULTIMATE BOOK OF
CBD REMEDIES

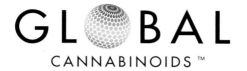

GLOBAL
CANNABINOIDS ™

THE ULTIMATE BOOK OF
CBD REMEDIES

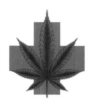

LEADING EXPERTS EXPLAIN
WHAT WORKS, WHAT DOESN'T, AND HOW
CBD IS CHANGING THE WORLD

RYAN LEWIS
CEO OF GLOBAL CANNABINOIDS™
Foreword by TRACY RYAN

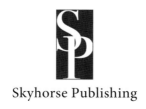

Skyhorse Publishing

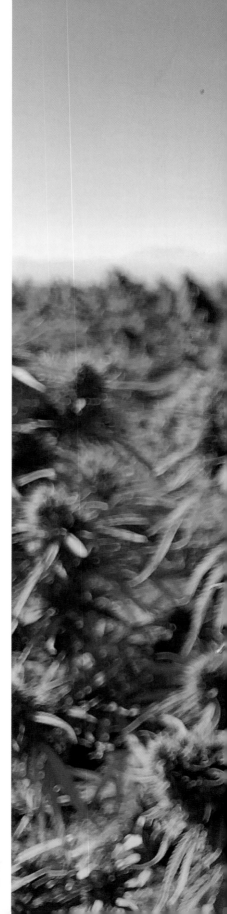

Skyhorse Publishing books may be purchased in bulk at special discounts for sales promotion, corporate gifts, fund-raising, or educational purposes. Special editions can also be created to specifications. For details, contact the Special Sales Department, Skyhorse Publishing, 307 West 36th Street, 11th Floor, New York, NY 10018 or info@skyhorsepublishing.com.

Skyhorse® and Skyhorse Publishing® are registered trademarks of Skyhorse Publishing, Inc.®, a Delaware corporation.

Visit our website at www.skyhorsepublishing.com.

10 9 8 7 6 5 4 3 2 1

Library of Congress Cataloging-in-Publication Data is available on file.

Cover design by Brian Peterson

Print ISBN: 978-1-5107-5744-8
Ebook ISBN: 978-1-5107-5745-5

Printed in the United States of America

Flowering buds ready for harvest droop in the sun, heavy with promising chemical compounds like CBD.

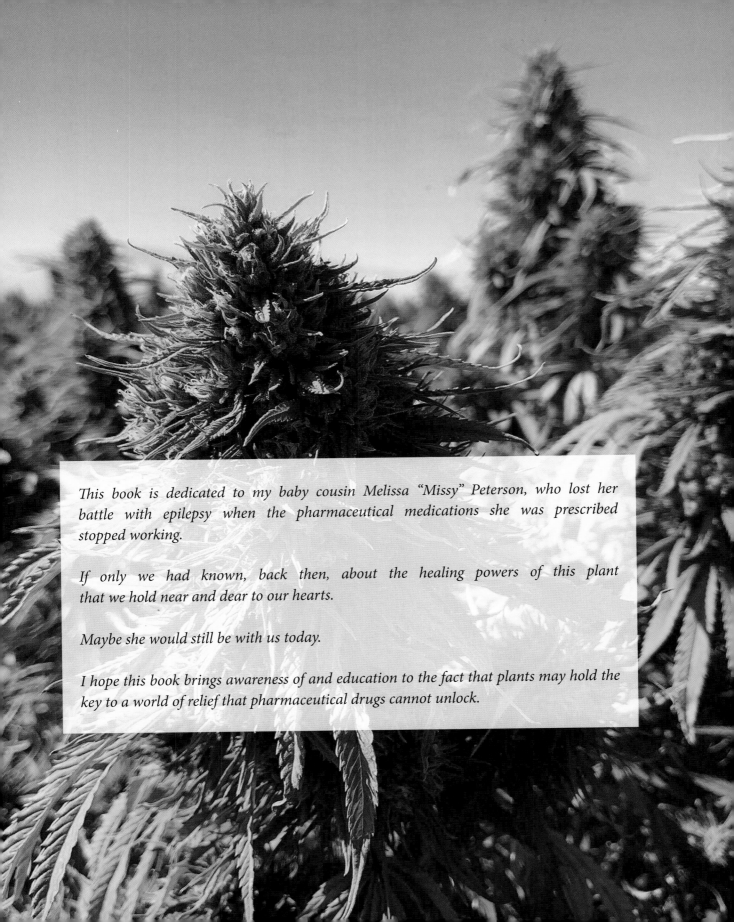

This book is dedicated to my baby cousin Melissa "Missy" Peterson, who lost her battle with epilepsy when the pharmaceutical medications she was prescribed stopped working.

If only we had known, back then, about the healing powers of this plant that we hold near and dear to our hearts.

Maybe she would still be with us today.

I hope this book brings awareness of and education to the fact that plants may hold the key to a world of relief that pharmaceutical drugs cannot unlock.

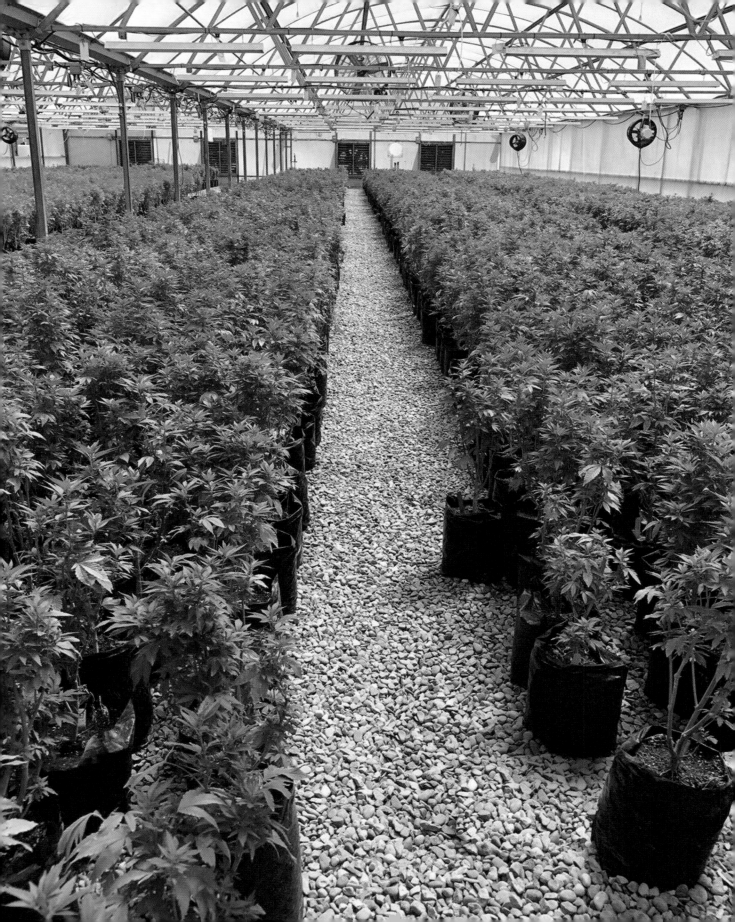

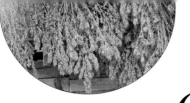
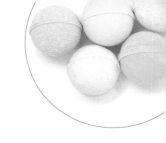

CONTENTS

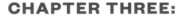
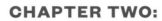
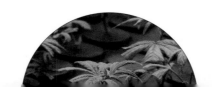
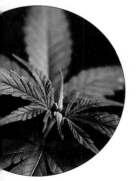
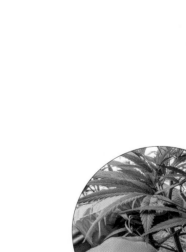

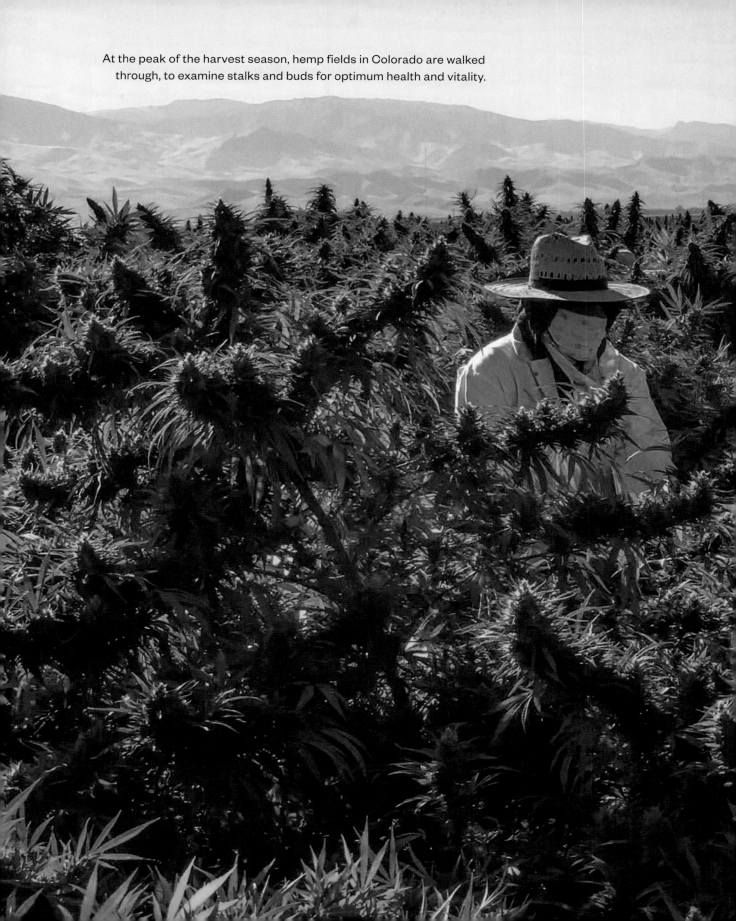

At the peak of the harvest season, hemp fields in Colorado are walked through, to examine stalks and buds for optimum health and vitality.

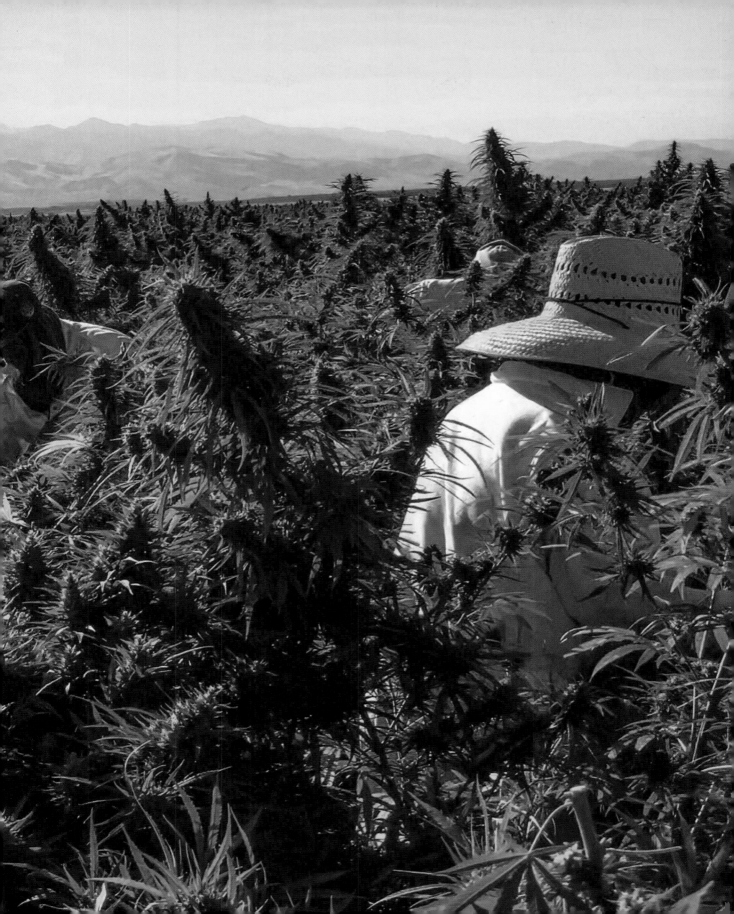

PREFACE

I wanted to write this book because I saw a genuine need for honest and credible information regarding cannabis, from people who were tired of suffering from a lack of solutions and wanted to be better informed and more in control of their options regarding health and well-being. Over the years I have seen an increasing dependence on pharmaceutical drugs, some of which fail to address the root issues of many of the diseases and general discomforts that they seek to treat, while simultaneously creating harmful and sometimes deadly side effects—like what we have seen with opioid epidemic.

Most people are either familiar with—or know someone familiar—losing a close one because of the fallible nature of doctors or an undesired result from prescription drugs. When my cousin Missy died from epilepsy, I saw first-hand the failure of pharmaceuticals—and in that moment I knew I wanted to do everything in my power to prevent other families from going through such a heart wrenching breach of trust in modern medicine. There had to be a better way . . . something that was waiting to be unlocked and explored . . . that we just hadn't discovered yet.

My journey to hemp, CBD, and the endocannabinoid system had begun.

The journey of cannabis itself originated thousands of years ago, perhaps longer than many of us could speculate, with many revelations along the way. The hurdles and, interestingly enough, achievements happened because of intentional misinformation and could have been dispelled multiple times using clinical research which, unfortunately, was halted abruptly after the first official trial around 1940. Fast forward to modern times where we are seeing that it is now *our* responsibility to find the truth, using new legislation and the power of communities who want to make an impact on debilitating and sometimes life-threatening diseases like cancer, epilepsy, autism, and inflammation using hemp cannabinoids. I wanted this book to be a companion, if you will, on this evolution we are experiencing in re-discovering cannabis—specifically CBD—because I feel that we truly are on the edge of a brand new world of well-being. In a society where we have every "answer" at our fingertips, it is still mind blowing to consider how much time we would need to invest into understanding the truth behind something as complex as the cannabis plant. With over a hundred chemical compounds, the research and clinical studies we have begun conducting on cannabis and cannabinoids (like CBD) barely even scratches the surface of what this plant is and could be capable of, both in humans and animals.

I have seen and personally witnessed people who had lost hope of ever feeling better, as a result of being unsuccessfully treated by pharmaceuticals for symptoms that were thought to be "untreatable," completely turn their lives around by using hemp cannabinoids. To not only improve from the use of naturally occurring compounds like CBD, but often heal completely. I realize that's a bold

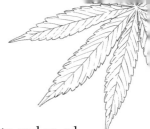

statement, but it is a truth for me, and I am hoping that you will be able to see that it is indeed true.

Throughout this book I have tried to not only detail some of these amazing stories of recovery and healing for you, but to also offer the science that goes along with it, as well as thoughts and ideas from leading experts, showing why and how cannabinoids like CBD do what they do. Working with these respected individuals and compiling the information contained within will re-formulate and re-educate how people perceive this often misrepresented plant so that everyone—especially the children suffering from cancer and other terminal illnesses—will find the well deserved peace they seek.

Ryan Lewis
March 2020

All proceeds from the sales of this book will be donated to www.savingsophie.org, which is a nonprofit organization focused on providing resources to families who are afflicted by pediatric and adult cancer, autism, or epilepsy, as well as supporting the scientists who are working towards creating less toxic treatments.

FOREWORD
BY TRACY RYAN

If you had told me, eight years ago, that I would be purposefully giving CBD or THC products to children, I would've told you to stop smoking so much of it! But that is exactly what has transpired. My husband, Josh, and I were just like most of the world at that time. Stigmatized by decades of lies and propaganda that the government has been feeding us about the dangers of this very medicinal herb.

It all started when our daughter, Sophie, was diagnosed seven years ago with a low-grade brain tumor at just eight and a half months old. Her tumor is considered a survivable one with an over 90 percent survival rate, but one that recurs frequently, with an 85 percent recurrence rate, and chemo being the only option.

The devastation was unlike anything either of us had ever experienced. When we learned that only 3.8 percent of all government funding goes to pediatric cancer research, and that only four new drugs had been brought to market in forty years for kids, the shock from it all was almost too much to bear. How could this even be true? We didn't have cell phones forty years ago. How could there be such a lack of science for our children??

After being connected to Ricki Lake and Abby Epstein through a random chain of events on social media, just days after Sophie's diagnosis, they informed me of the documentary they had just begun filming that is now on Netflix called *Weed the People*. After much discussion and being surrounded by teams of experts, we made the choice to explore cannabis as medicine. This wasn't a decision we took lightly. It came after Josh and I completed hours and hours of research and consulted with Sophie's oncologists, who all agreed to try the medicinal oils on our baby.

Sophie took her first dose of cannabis, containing all of the cannabinoids that naturally occur in the plant, at just nine months old . . . on camera.

Multiple surgeries have been successfully performed on Sophie's brain tumor, using hemp cannabinoids to bolster and strengthen her immune system.

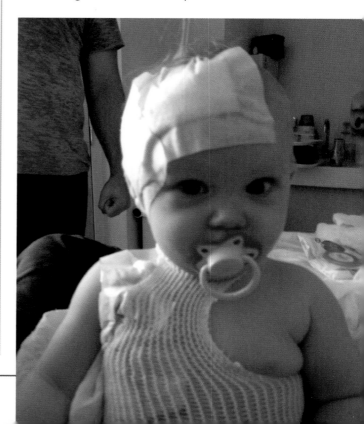

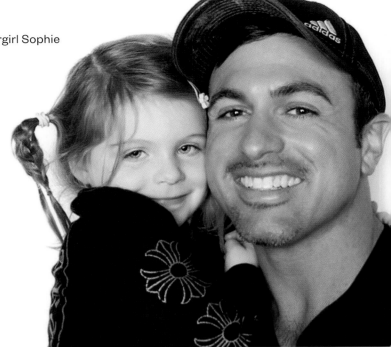

Ryan Lewis and Cannakid Supergirl Sophie

What we have witnessed in our own child, and thousands of other adults and children worldwide over the last several years, has been simply astonishing. To see what this plant is capable of is unlike anything I have ever witnessed. Treating cancer, epilepsy, autism, PTSD, MS, fibromyalgia, chronic/cevere pain, and beyond. There are many lives that have been lost unnecessarily and lives that could have been changed dramatically, if only cannabinoids had been utilized. So we made the decision to try and do something about it.

A year into chemo with Sophie, we were absolutely convinced that we had to do more to help people become familiar with how this plant can be used. We started our own company, which we named "CannaKids," that is now a provider of a medical cannabis tincture brand in California as well as our 501c3 charity SavingSophie.org. We wanted to give patients access to this medicine, education, and financial support.

So, our journey began.

It was through the support of Ryan Lewis, and the incredible CBD oils he gave us access to, that contributed to how we effectively helped thousands upon thousands of patients. The partnership that we forged turned into a friendship that has been one of my most valued in the entire industry. Ryan consistently puts our family and our patients first . . . so to be able to support this book for him is truly an honor.

People have come from all over the world to California in order to get access to our products. Successes were so profound that they have led us to groundbreaking clinical trials with a world renowned-cancer research scientist, Dr. Anahid Jewett. And findings that we feel confident will help us not only legalize this plant, but guide us into a new age of how diseases are treated.

Now two years later, after studys of seventeen of our CannaKids patients in varying stages of disease, both young and old, the discoveries just keep coming. We have found that cannabis attacks and kills cancer stem cells, which chemo and radiation can't even do. It also turns the NK Cell system back to when it was otherwise in a state of malfunction. The very system that protects us from cancer in the first place.

This has been a nonstop roller coaster of highs and lows for a very long seven years. But we are now working our way toward human trials with nontoxic therapeutics, which we believe will revolutionize medicine.

It's people like Ryan, and the bravery of

patients like our daughter, that have allowed us to be so successful in bringing this plant to the masses . . . and we won't stop until there is access for all! If you have picked up this book, we applaud you! Welcome to the world of natural healing, through cannabis.

Baby Sophie with her mom, CannaKids founder Tracy Ryan

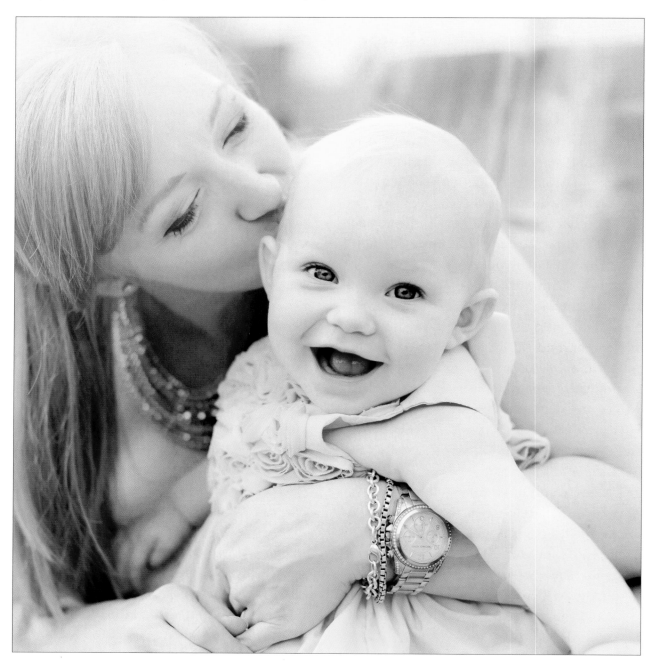

INTRODUCTION

CBD (cannabidiol) is one of the most important medical and nutritional innovations of the twenty-first century. It's been used safely for literally thousands of years, yet we are only just now unlocking its true potential. As the founder of one of the world's largest bulk and wholesale cannabinoid distribution platform—GlobalCannabinoids. io—I've had a front-row seat for the multiple breakthroughs that CBD has experienced in the past decade, and also for the exciting innovations that are driving this product's explosive growth across platforms. When it comes to CBD, it is no exaggeration to say that the breakthroughs that change how we understand CBD are coming on a near-daily basis! From medicine to skin care to personal care and beyond, CBD is poised to positively impact multiple aspects of our lives in the coming years. For some users, these impacts may be relatively small (such as greater ease in falling asleep, or pleasant and beneficial cosmetic effects). But for others, CBD stands to be absolutely life-changing.

There is tangible excitement to be felt when one is standing at the beginning of a revolution. These days, there is a growing number of people who feel that this is precisely where we are in the world of hemp cannabinoids. Each year, the funding for research into CBD expands. Physicians are choosing to become more educated about the benefits of

hemp cannabinoids like CBD and are able to discuss treatment options with their patients. As an industry, hemp cannabinoids have expanded beyond a subset of "cannabis culture" to find a mainstream acceptance with CBD that now rivals any other supplements in the marketplace.

At the same time, CBD isn't quite there yet. We still have a way to go, and I think we're currently in a period of transition, because more and more people are discovering CBD every day and I believe it's important to let research and facts guide our narrative. We need to guard against disinformation, exaggeration, and people just stopping by to make a buck—problems every new breakthrough faces but that especially plague the hemp community—and let the medicine that exists in the hemp plant speak for itself. There's so much clinical research pointing to the effectiveness of CBD in a wide range of conditions that we don't need to embellish . . . we need to explore. Breaking down what is fact and what is fiction—and what is yet to be discovered about hemp—is an important reason why I wanted to write this book.

I'm the kind of person who thinks that when consumers have all the information presented to them clearly, they will make sensible choices. That's why I believe that, sooner or later, most American consumers are bound to embrace the benefits that hemp cannabinoids,

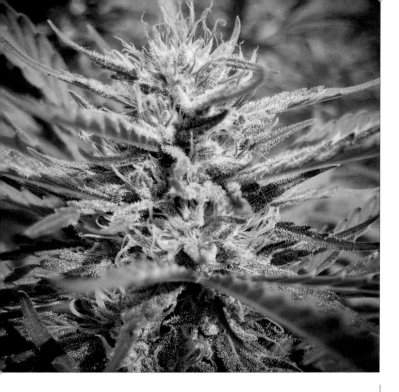

like CBD, have to offer. If we can look past the long-debunked stereotypes and mistaken associations linking hemp to a singular cannabinoid (THC) that has mind-altering effects and look to the real, hard science—that hemp/cannabis has over 100 cannabinoids with medicinal value like CBD—then maybe hemp can finally obtain the status it deserves, an amazing plant that is truly crucial for maintaining and improving health.

To cut right to the chase, the fictions about hemp/cannabis—and the hesitations that keep some consumers from educating themselves about it further—tend to stem from the fact that all hemp cannabinoids, like CBD, are from a cannabis plant. It is Cannabis Sativa, bred to have higher levels of certain cannabinoids like CBD. I don't think there's any good reason to skirt around this point. Instead, I say let's tackle it head-on! The more people know about where CBD comes from, how it is derived, and what it can do, the more

people will be willing to take the next step into improving the quality of their lives. Like we said, there are over one hundred natural chemical compounds, or "cannabinoids," occurring in the hemp (or cannabis/marijuana) plant. Most consumers are aware that Tetrahydrocannabinol—or THC—is one of these cannabinoids and that it produces the "high" people feel when they use cannabis. Many people associate hemp or cannabis with the "high" feeling, when in all reality, hemp is much more . . . as we are now learning with CBD. It's true that both CBD and THC are found in cannabis, and both have a three-letter abbreviation, but the similarities stop there! CBD is *not* psychoactive and produces *no* narcotic effect at all. You'll never "feel high" by using it, no matter how much you take. CBD is in no way mind-altering and does not impair its users.

However, what it *does* do is decrease the amount of inflammation and cortisol in the body, which relieves anxiety, eases pain, relieves symptoms associated with the nervous system, the digestive system, and the immune system, and provides relief from irritating skin conditions. Less tangibly—but just as important—millions of users say it simply makes them feel better! And it does all of this while being extremely safe and nonaddictive. Side effects linked to CBD are almost unheard of yet tend to include things like mild headaches or nausea upon ingestion. This usually happens when the endocannabinoid system (don't worry, we will get to that) inside our bodies has never been activated before. Best of all, because of the nature of its chemical composition and function, the human body does not grow accustomed to CBD—meaning that longtime users never need to "up their dose" to get the same effect they experienced when starting their treatment. Instead, CBD's benefits stay consistent because the job of the endocannabinoid system is to create and maintain homeostasis.

One of the reasons I like being in the hemp business is that I get to be on the "leading edge" of all the explosive changes in the marketplace. New discoveries and innovation are driving the development of new products and remedies, which use hemp cannabinoids like CBD, at a dizzying pace. I can tell you from firsthand experience: if you want to work in an industry with zero excitement and a slow rate of change, don't go into hemp cannabinoids! But for those of you in this space already, just know that while many Americans have yet to try CBD—or even to fully understand what it is—there are also millions who love what they have already discovered, and, just like you, they understand what a great thing this can be for people who are suffering from things that are currently untreatable with modern medicine. They know it, they like it, and they want more.

According to Forbes, CBD sales are expected to hit $20 billion by 2024, increasing as much as 700 percent in the year 2020. Clearly, that cat is out of the bag. *Someone* has discovered the positive effects of CBD, and more and more people are learning about its benefits in an effort to take control of their health in a natural way. As I'll try to make clear

in this book, that's a *very* good thing—not just for me, but for the medicinal community as a whole and the thousands of patients who are still searching for relief from symptoms that modern treatments can't seem to manage. I've sometimes been called a "crusader for hemp." I'm not sure how I feel about that title, but I suppose there are different ways you can interpret it. I don't think I'm a "crusader" if that means blindly following a cause, no matter what. (As I'll emphasize again and again in this book, the evidence for hemp cannabinoids like CBD, is so strong that we don't need to exaggerate its effectiveness.) With that said, if people mean that I want to advocate for bringing the restorative capacities of CBD to as many people as possible . . . then go ahead and call me a crusader.

If you're new to cannabinoids like CBD, and are a little bit skeptical as to some of the claims you've heard, that's OK! I'm here to win you over the right way—using peer-reviewed studies, data, and science . . . in addition to the compelling anecdotal stories about how hemp has improved people's lives, literally all over the world.

If you're reading this book and you *already* have a good knowledge of CBD, you might be wondering why it needs an advocate at all. On the one hand, I'd say that you're right. Hemp doesn't need anyone to brag about what it can do; it can speak for itself. However, it does need someone to clearly outline the truth of its ability to change lives. Each day, people using CBD for the first time are becoming evangelists for it. (As "one guy" in the CBD industry, it's probably beyond my power to add to or detract from this effect!)

But on the other hand, there are unfortunately still forces that would like to see CBD adoption delayed as long as possible (if not permanently). Because of these forces, we need to make sure that we present all the facts regarding hemp and specifically CBD in the right way.

I think some of the resistance to CBD comes from people who may be well intentioned, but are simply misinformed about what it is and what it does. These folks can be converted . . . given time, of course. But there are also powerful, moneyed interests in the establishment that are going to push against CBD tooth and nail precisely because it *does* work so well . . . and across such a broad spectrum. Into this group I would place pharmaceutical companies currently selling medicines that do not work as well as CBD, on the conditions they are intended to treat, that carry a whole host of side effects that CBD does not. (Accessing traditional pharmaceuticals can also involve negotiating unaffordable premium costs and a whole host of other hidden costs involved in the healthcare industry, while CBD presents a more accessible and more effective alternative.) There are cosmetics companies that would prefer to sell consumers makeup and creams that give skin the *appearance* of health, while CBD can genuinely eliminate blemishes and give users evenly toned, glowing, healthy skin. These and other businesses will do everything in their power to discredit CBD,

spread misconceptions about it, and convince consumers that it's not something they want to get involved in.

Entities like private prisons and law enforcement can have a direct interest in ensuring that cannabinoids remain illegal.

And I can't let that happen.

I can't because millions of people—right now, all across the country—are experiencing pain that I know CBD can cure. They have health issues of all sizes that CBD can address. Some will use it to feel less anxious, sleep better, and reduce inflammation. Some will use it to correct more serious health issues. But whether someone's issue is large or small, if a hemp cannabinoid like CBD can fix it, then I'm going to try to make that happen—and I'm confident that the thousands of other advocates for CBD across the country are going to help, as well.

This brings me to another issue CBD currently faces, which I feel I should note in the introduction so I don't lose anyone. I call it: "What's the catch?"

Put plainly, the ever-expanding list of things that hard science is proving CBD can do is just too much for some people to believe. I don't blame anybody for having a healthy skepticism, especially when it comes to claims about products that can improve your health and appearance. We're all familiar with supplements that haven't lived up to their advertising claims. We've all seen claims about classes, or home gyms, or other self-improvement programs that were too good to be true. (I don't blame consumers for being skeptical. America has a history of hucksters telling tall tales!)

But in our long history, we've *also* seen advancements like penicillin. Like sterilization and pasteurization. Like medical imaging technology and immunotherapy. We've seen innovations that *did* live up to the hype and provided a benefit to society so deep and profound that we wondered how we'd ever gotten along without them.

In short, sometimes advances and discoveries are *not* too good to be true. They're simply true. They can improve our lives in dramatic ways and carry no significant downside or trade-off. I believe that CBD falls squarely into this category. Why? Because of the endocannabinoid system that exists within *all* mammals. Cannabis is made for us.

With its wide range of application, hemp/cannabis and more specifically CBD have the potential to impact a large percentage of the population. Because of the variability of its effects—which are being researched by top minds around the world at this very moment—it has the potential to do a lot of good for general well-being, and for a select few its benefits will be absolutely life-changing. Its lack of potential for abuse or addiction, and its multiple delivery systems, mean that many people can start to benefit from using hemp cannabinoids immediately.

In this book, I'll provide a guide to the research on CBD that has already been done, the ongoing discoveries and their potential, and the questions we need to ask to prepare for the future. We'll cover the most serious conditions that CBD holds the potential to treat and include perspectives from leading medical experts. We'll also look at the "innovators" in this space who have been researching and studying cannabinoids like CBD for decades. We'll try to answer questions like "Who is conducting the best research?" "Who stands to benefit from advances in CBD, and how?" And, most importantly, "Who can we trust to provide impartial information on this revolutionary plant compound?"

In addition, I'll lay out the practical steps to help ensure you're accessing the best possible CBD products—and the most appropriate products for the condition(s) you are trying to treat. We'll look at the different ways consumers use CBD, and how to figure out the kind of CBD delivery method that might work best for you. I'll try to answer the most common questions people have about CBD. (And trust me: when it comes to CBD, there *are* no silly questions.) I'll also provide more than a little "insider's perspective" on what I think the future holds, and where I personally think CBD treatments are headed.

There's no question that we're living in a revolutionary time when it comes to medicine and technology. Historians hundreds of years from now are bound to find this period notable for its rapid advancements. Some of these advances come from new scientific discoveries and innovations, but other light-bulb moments come from looking at something that's been around for thousands of years . .

. and seeing it in a new way. Time and again, we are finding that cures and breakthroughs lie all around us, but we're only now able to understand and access them.

Humans have been enjoying the benefits of hemp for thousands of years, both medicinally and with use in textiles, yet it has been purposely and solely associated with the "high feeling" due to the interconnected cannabinoids like THC. That ends here. That ends now.

In the twenty-first century, we've finally "cracked the code" to understand the awesome potential of hemp cannabinoids like CBD as medicine that can stand on its own. And, in my opinion, the most exciting thing about all of this is that we are just getting started. The journey into the future of hemp and CBD is going to be an exciting and dramatic one.

I hope I can convince you to come along for the ride.

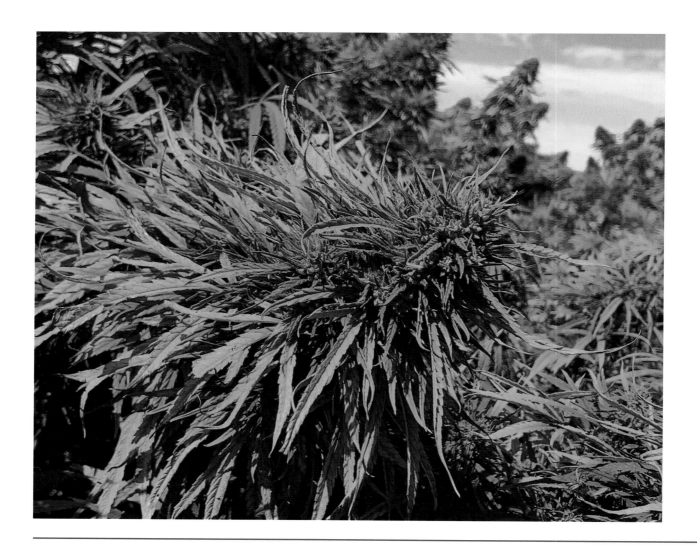

CHAPTER ONE
THE JOURNEY TO CBD

Revolutions do not come out of nowhere. They do not occur spontaneously. Rather, they are the result of forces that have been at play for years—sometimes generations—often working behind the scenes. They are the result of embers carefully tended. Then when the moment is right—or the technology becomes advanced enough—they can ignite to usher forth great change. The story of CBD is an excellent example of how a long and winding road can lead to a revolution.

Humans have used cannabis for millennia, and this meant being subject to all the cannabinoids in cannabis, most notably THC. People who used cannabis found that they felt a pleasant "high" as well as a reduction in their

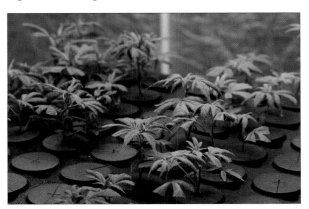

Tiny sproutlings are lovingly tended and fortified so they can thrive in fields where they will often reach twenty times the height shown here.

pain. Many of them felt other pleasant effects, as well. Anyone could be forgiven for assuming that these effects were all one in the same, and not the result of a multitude of individual cannabinoids, each with their own properties, working synergistically with the body.

While THC provides an intoxicating high, it is CBD that gives cannabis users their cessation of pain. CBD and THC are different from each other in many other respects, as well.

I think a great first step to understanding the difference between CBD and THC—and what makes CBD so revolutionary—is to understand how these substances interact with our bodies when we use them.

THE ENDOCANNABINOID SYSTEM

Ahhh, the ECS. The endocannabinoid system is what allows CBD—and the other cannabinoids naturally occurring in hemp—to return our bodies to homeostasis. It's hard to fully understand how hemp cannabinoids like CBD work without getting a basic grasp of the endocannabinoid system. (Otherwise, it's a bit like trying to understand how a record is played, yet never examining a record player.)

The endocannabinoid system (or ECS) is a

neural system in your body comprised of neurotransmitters that bind to cannabinoid receptors in your central nervous system. Before we go any further, I must clearly state that the endocannabinoid system has some of the most prominent neurotransmitters in the body—all over the body—and should have been taught to us right alongside the cardiovascular system. It is a major system in the body, a lot like a conductor in an orchestra.

The receptors are present in your brain, and also in the more peripheral parts of your central nervous system. The endocannabinoid system is still being studied, but scientists believe it is very much involved in the regulation of things like pain, mood, and cognitive processes. This system processes and manifests the pharmacological effects of cannabis when humans use it (or an extract from it).

The endocannabinoid system includes three basic components that help it do what it does.

The first of these is endogenous arachidonate-based lipids such as anandamide. Naturally produced by the body, anandamide's name is taken from a Sanskrit word which means "bliss and delight." That should give you a good clue as to its function! First discovered and named in 1992 by Dr. Raphael Mechoulam (look for more on him later), anandamide is a fatty acid neurotransmitter that impacts the central nervous system and the peripheral nervous system. Anandamide has been shown to govern things like memory, feeding behavior, and pleasure. Its receptors are sensitive to the psychoactive ingredient in cannabis, THC.

The second component of the endocannabinoid system are the enzymes that synthesize and degrade endocannabinoids. One example of these enzymes would be fatty acid amide hydrolase. This substance is shown to break down anandamide in humans. Because it is closely tied to the regulation of feelings like fear, pain, and anxiety, it is currently the subject of considerable scientific study. Another example of these enzymes is monoacylglyerol lipase.

The third component of the endocannabinoid system includes

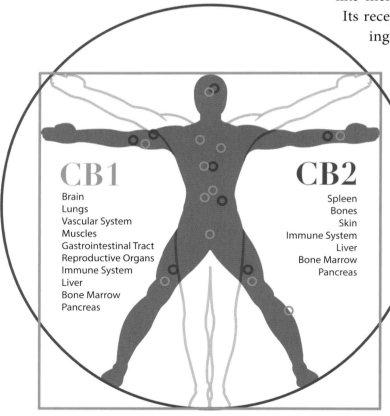

CB1

Brain
Lungs
Vascular System
Muscles
Gastrointestinal Tract
Reproductive Organs
Immune System
Liver
Bone Marrow
Pancreas

CB2

Spleen
Bones
Skin
Immune System
Liver
Bone Marrow
Pancreas

the cannabinoid receptors CB1 and CB2. CB1 is receptive to compounds found in THC, but its primary activator is anandamide. CB2 is closely related to CB1 but is found to regulate inflammation, irritation, and similar reactions. CB1 receptors are most commonly found in the central nervous system and in major tissues and organs. In contrast, CB2 reception tends to be located in the peripheral nervous system and GI tract, though it can be found in other locations, as well. There are many parts of the body where you'll find both CB1 and CB2 receptors. However, note that CBD doesn't directly trigger CB1 or CB2. Instead, it modifies the ability of CB1 and CB2 to bind to cannabinoids. CBD also impacts the ECS by enhancing the body's natural levels of endocannabinoids.

As you might imagine, the ECS's connection to our brains is very powerful. Both CB1 and CB2 are found within the brain, and the ECS has the power to stimulate the brain to regulate things like stress, mood, anxiety, and pleasure.

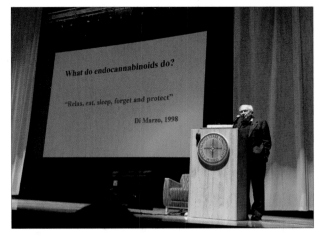

Raphael Mechoulam explaining a quote regarding the potential of cannabinoids in everyday well-being.

It is also connected to the parts of the brain that can sometimes be impacted by neurological diseases like epilepsy and Alzheimer's.

The study of the ECS and the study of cannabinoids have always been closely connected. In 1964, researchers first isolated the psychoactive ingredient of cannabis, THC. You might say that the isolation of THC gave the scientific community enough to focus on. There was no call to quickly move to other components of cannabis (such as CBD). In fact, many scientists assumed that THC was entirely responsible for the salutary effects that cannabis users reported.

THC is a lipid. Biologists believe that the cannabis plant evolved it as a defensive measure against being eaten by predators, against UV light, and possibly against environmental stress. For many years, scientists thought they understood how THC worked when it produced its "high" effects on users. However, it turned out that they had more to learn. Scientists knew that cannabis and THC functioned thanks to a cellular receptor (present in all humans, on the surface of cells in many parts of the body). Scientists understood that when someone used cannabis—such as by smoking marijuana—the THC would bind to CB1 sites to produce a number of sensations (many of them desirable). Yet scientists were initially wrong in one major conjecture: they believed that CB1 receptors could *only* interact with THC molecules—that they were "custom built" to receive THC. But that wasn't the case. As research continued, scientists found that CB1 receptors could also accommodate a number of other molecules.

At the same time, researchers also came to

How Cannabis Works

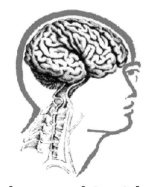

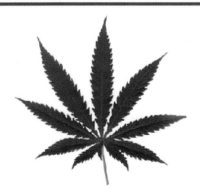

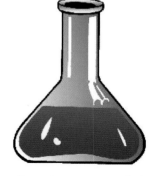

Endocannabinoids (Brain Derived)	**Phytocannabinoids (Plant Derived)**	**Synthetic Cannabinoids (Pharmaceutical Lab)**
Foods: Omega-3s & Omega-6s	Buds, Tinctures, Extracts	Patented Synthesized Compound
Anandamide (AEA)	THC, CBD, CBN, etc.	THC-only (Marinol)

Endocannabinoid Receptors (Brain Receptors)

CB1, CB2, etc.

The endocannabinoid system (ECS) is involved in regulating a variety of physiological processes including appetite, pain and pleasure sensation, immune system, mood, and memory.

Image Credit: pinterest.com

understand the importance of CB2 receptors. Unlike CB1 receptors, CB2 receptors directly impact our ability to manage afflictions like inflammatory diseases, autoimmune diseases, bowel diseases, arthritis, and allergies.

Even before there was talk of simply incorporating THC into medicine, scientists were looking for ways to harness these receptor interactions.

In the 1980s, pharmaceutical giant Eli

Lilly developed a "synthetic THC" drug called Nabilone, which was aimed at combating pain and nausea. While it did have some positive effects, the drug never caught on. This may have been because of its side effects, which could include substantial disorientation and dizziness. One study even found that Nabilone could *increase* pain when it was given to post-operative patients. (Because of these setbacks, Lilly ceased efforts to get the drug approved in the 1980s. However, it was later acquired by Valeant Pharmaceuticals, which eventually received FDA approval in 2006. Today, it is used to treat chemotherapy-related vomiting, fibromyalgia, and PTSD.)

Despite early disappointments, like Nabilone, research into cannabinoid receptors (and medicines to act on them) continued. As it did, new worlds related to CB1 and CB2 slowly began to open up. Scientists began looking more closely at the hundreds of other compounds that were able to interact with CB1 and CB2—including CBD. No longer simply a receptor for THC, CB1 was now understood to be a gateway for a whole host of interactions with different functions throughout the body.

By the early 1990s, researchers studying cannabis had identified even more counterparts to THC also present in cannabis. They collectively termed them endocannabinoids. N-arachidonoylethanolamine (anandamide, AEA) was discovered in 1992, and 2-arachidonoylglycerol (2-AG) was discovered in 1995. This additional research shed more light on the endocannabinoid system (ECS) and how

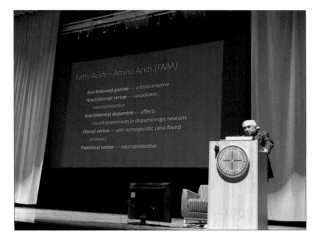

Raphael Mechoulam details some of the essential fatty acids involved in hemp cannabinoid assimilation.

it might hold keys to impacting our well-being and health. It was these innovations that laid the groundwork for much of the CBD research (and research into other cannabinoids) being undertaken today.

This is a very short primer on the endocannabinoid system, but many online resources exist if you're interested in taking a "deep dive" and really understanding the nuances of its inner workings on a granular level.

It was important for the scientific community to discover the endocannabinoid system, and to grasp the basics of which constituent parts of cannabis acted upon it. However, the story of cannabis and CBD in the United States is not a strictly scientific one. I believe to understand how we got where we are today, it is also useful to frame the political, social, and legal history of cannabis products. As you will see, they are all much older than the country itself!

CANNABIS IN THE UNITED STATES

The first evidence of human interaction with hemp goes back thousands of years. (Historians aren't exactly sure when humans first began foraging for and/or growing hemp/cannabis. Some have put it as far back as 12,000 years ago. Others estimate that it's closer to 3,000 years.) However, to understand the relationship between humans and hemp, it's important to note the relationship between cannabis and hemp.

In case the terms are unfamiliar to you, hemp is a *kind* of cannabis, one of three different varieties. What makes hemp special is that

1. It is incredibly useful for making things;
2. like other strains of cannabis, it can be bred to contain very high levels of CBD, CBC, CBN, and other beneficial cannabinoids that can bring balance, relief, and healing to our bodies; and
3. the THC content is very low, making it extremely difficult or impossible to use hemp for the purpose of getting high.

In the ancient world, hemp emerged as a prominent fiber for use in all kinds of products. During certain periods of global history, hemp was one of the most cultivated crops on the planet! Even today, many cultures still grow hemp primarily for its textile purposes.

At the same time, the earliest uses of hemp for medicinal purposes emerged in 2000 BC in India, where it was cultivated for internal use to treat illnesses of varying types. From there, word of its efficacy slowly traveled around the globe. By the year 100 or so, it had shown up in what we would today call "traditional Chinese medicine" as a cure for pain. (It is somewhat opaque as to where "medicinal uses" and "recreational uses" blended into each other in the ancient world.)

In the Early and Late Middle Ages, hemp remained a dominant material for making things like rope, sails on ships, and clothing. Then, with the emergence of the printing press, hemp-based paper became extremely popular. During this same period, several scientists and physicians of the day started to study the properties of cannabis (including hemp) in an attempt to verify some of the claims made about it. Some of these physicians deduced that cannabis held the ability to cure a wide variety of diseases and conditions. (I tend to be skeptical of the findings of these doctors, but some of the things that medieval physicians claimed cannabis could do—such as treat inflammation and discomfort—*are*, I must admit, among the same things we'd say it can do today)

By the time Columbus sailed for the "New World," hemp was already a staple of the European economy. At various times, Italy, Russia, and other nations took turns being the "hemp powerhouse" of their day. European countries realized that hemp was important and planned to cultivate it in the lands they

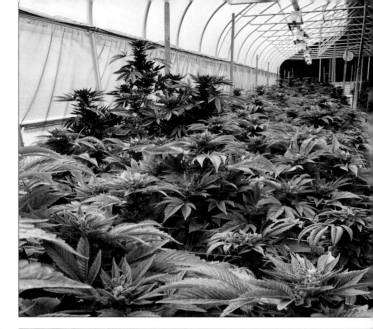

began conquering and claiming. Before it was ever cultivated in North America, the Spanish were growing hemp in what would one day be Chile.

In the 1600s, records show that British subjects grew hemp in Virginia for export back to England. (This is the very first report of cannabis being cultivated in what would become the United States.) This hemp was generally used for making rope. As the years went by, many prominent colonial-era Americans (not just George Washington) grew industrial hemp.

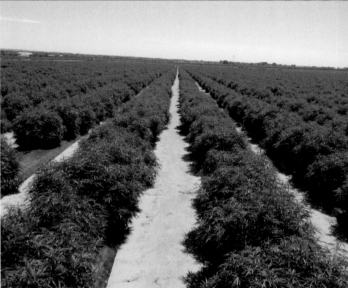

Throughout the 1700s, there was no general awareness in the United States that hemp belonged to a family of plants that could produce psychoactive, medicinal, and/or healing effects. However, that began to change in the 1800s, when Irish physician William Brooke O'Shaughnessy began conducting research on the medicinal effects of cannabis. His findings were printed in popular and academic journals of the day, and an interest in cannabis as medicine began to grow. By the 1850s, pharmacies and physicians in the United States began to offer cannabis and cannabis extracts in various forms.

At around the same time, a market for recreational use also began to emerge. In cities like New York, Boston, and Chicago, parlors opened where customers could partake of cannabis, alongside opium and other drugs. Some of these establishments were located in "vice neighborhoods"—such as Chicago's infamous Levee District—where cannabis-selling

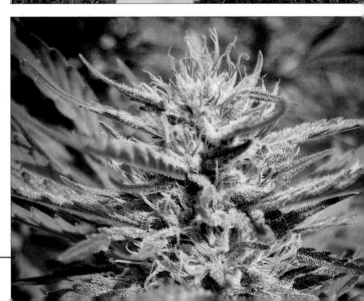

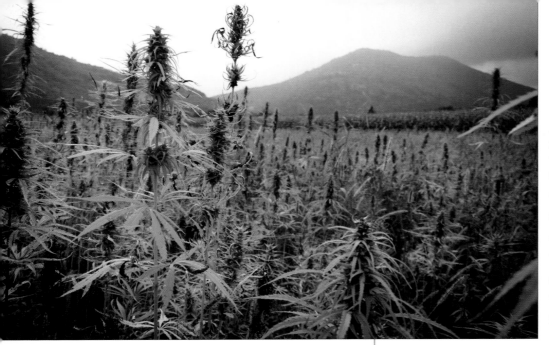

In their early months, hemp flowers enjoy drinking in the morning mists.

establishments sat side by side with brothels, casinos, and bars. However, in some cities—such as Boston, for example—accounts exist of cannabis establishments targeting upper-class customers in the city's tonier neighborhoods.

Hemp and cannabis, for a time, became a visible and open part of American culture. Hemp was an important crop used to make many useful things, and recreational cannabis was increasingly easy to find in urban areas. Until the year 1900, the reverse side of a $10 bill even portrayed hemp farming.

Yet as the use of cannabis had grown in the years after the Civil War, there came to be increased interest in regulating it. By the early twentieth century, this regulation began to take serious hold at the state level, with some laws passed requiring a physician's prescription for cannabis. Other states called for it to be labeled to warn consumers of its potential potency, while additional ones passed legislation to have it categorized as a known poison! (Oddly, most of these states still allowed cannabis to be sold to consumers but simply required that the bottle containing it be labeled POISON.)

The first national law to have a serious impact on cannabis was the Pure Food and Drug Act, passed by the federal government in 1906. The stated goal of the Act was to fight mislabeling of products and allow the government to crack down on fraudulent producers that sold food that did not contain the ingredients stated on their packaging. However, the Act also mandated that all products containing substances deemed by the government to be potentially dangerous—alcohol, cannabis, morphine, and opium among them—would be required to list them on the packaging. These substances were not made illegal, however. Even so, it caused many food and drug producers to change the ingredients they used. (For example, many historians believe Coca-Cola's decision to switch its active ingredient from cocaine to caffeine in 1903 was done in anticipation of the Act.) The Act also mandated that drug packaging contain dosing information to help consumers understand precisely how much they should take.

Some people saw the Pure Food and Drug

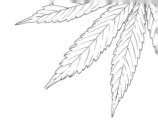

Act as a first step down the road to an outright ban on intoxicating substances, including cannabis. Others believed the opposite was true; they reasoned that since the federal government had shown *it* was going to "step up to the table" when it came to regulation, then states would no longer feel the need to ban or regulate these substances themselves. From this point of view, the Act might even usher in a new era of tolerance and permissiveness!

A few years after the Act was passed, it became clear that this interpretation was wishful thinking.

In 1911, Massachusetts passed additional laws to further regulate cannabis, and in 1914 New York and Maine followed suit. There was an increasing tendency of states to categorize cannabis as belonging to the class of habit-forming and addictive drugs from which consumers should be protected. California passed laws restricting cannabis and in 1914 conducted the first known cannabis "drug raid," confiscating a wagon filled with hemp in downtown Los Angeles. (Only a few newspaper clips reporting the historic drug raid still exist today. However, historians have established that there's strong evidence it was made by a largely Caucasian police force against hemp producers of Mexican origin. Entire books have been written about the selective enforcement of antidrug laws to target minority communities. I will merely note here that cannabis shares this troubling history, and it goes all the way back to the start of cannabis enforcement.)

In the fifteen years following the California raid, ten other US states passed laws restricting cannabis. Mexico went "whole hog" and made cannabis illegal in 1925. (Though the Harrison Act of 1914 imposed strict new drug laws that were enforced during this period, it was limited to drugs derived from "opium or coca leaves" and did not further regulate cannabis.)

Then, in 1930, the Federal Bureau of Narcotics was created by President Herbert Hoover. Functioning as a department of the United States Treasury, the FBN was inaugurated largely to respond to concerns over the importation of large quantities of opium to the United States from Southeast Asia. However, the FBN also enthusiastically investigated Americans illegally growing or consuming domestic cannabis. At the same time, some of these Americans pushed back, arguing that their cannabis was being grown or consumed without violating a specific state or federal law. This situation culminated in the passage of the Marijuana Tax Act of 1937 (sometimes spelled as "Marihuana Tax Act").

The Marijuana Tax Act did not criminalize the production of cannabis per se; it criminalized the production of cannabis without the paying of a new federal tax. It also imposed new taxes on physicians who prescribed cannabis, and pharmacists who sold it. Most domestic growers were content to pay the tax, though some resisted. (In one notable account, shortly after the Act's passage, two men—Samuel Caldwell and Moses Baca—were convicted of violating the Act. Caldwell

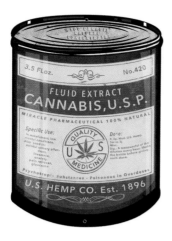 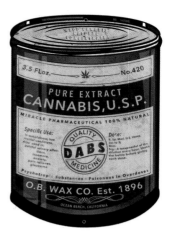

was sentenced to four years in jail, and Baca received eighteen months. They were the first men in US history ever to be convicted of federal cannabis crimes. Their relatively harsh sentences were meant to "send a message" that the government was serious about enforcement.)

The Marijuana Tax Act also had another important effect: it placed the term "marijuana" into the general public's lexicon for the first time. Though they might be familiar with hemp, most Americans had not heard the term "marijuana" before or, if they had, did not know what it referred to. (Of course, it didn't help the cause of cannabis that the very first time many Americans learned about marijuana was in a negative context.)

Many historians have pointed out that the Marijuana Tax Act did not seem to be especially needed at the time it was passed. Though Americans were struggling through the Great Depression—and the federal budget was under great strain—the revenue that stood to be collected from the Act was relatively modest. Moreover, there was no large-scale public outcry for the government to "do something about" cannabis producers. Cannabis cultivation and use was not associated with criminal activity, and cannabis was not generally viewed as a danger to users.

Thus, two other theories exist to explain why the Act was passed.

The first is that the FBN was simply seeking to grow its own budget. A new act to enforce would necessitate more agents, equipment, and funds. The FBN would have a basis to request all of these, and the agency itself would grow larger and more important. The second theory—which seems strange enough to have some truth to it—is that the Act was really aimed at hemp. A theory goes that a group of industrialists with links to the paper industry—among them, publishing tycoon William Randolph Hearst—was concerned that American-grown hemp would prove a cheaper and higher-quality alternative to the wood pulp currently used to print the nation's many newspapers. Hearst had just invested in massive holdings in timber, with an eye to vertical integration. But if the news industry were to transition to pulp made from hemp, his new business edge would be lost. Some believe that Hearst and his associates used their wealth and powerful political connections to see that the Marijuana Tax Act was passed.

Whether or not Hearst was actually behind the Act and its passage, the result must have pleased him. Hemp production in the United States remained relatively low—with a few producers still electing to pay the tax—and hemp never found a way to compete as a fiber for use in newspaper publishing.

But powerful as Hearst was, global geopolitical forces proved even more powerful in the years to come . . .

When the US joined the fight in World War II, the need suddenly arose to produce large amounts of rope and sails for the war effort. This needed to be done quickly and affordably. Suddenly, hemp was back on the table! More than that: to the astonishment of many, hemp soon became positively patriotic. The government immediately lifted any bans on hemp production (though obtaining a tax stamp was still required) and encouraged farmers to plant the crop in propaganda pieces. The most infamous of these—the short film *Hemp for Victory*—sought to tug on patriotic heartstrings by claiming that the USS *Constitution* had hemp sails, that the pioneers had ridden in Conestoga wagons featuring hemp coverings, and that hemp had been the original, authentically American fibrous plant grown by the nation's first farmers . . . before being pushed out by imported plans of "foreign" origin. Some of the claims in *Hemp for Victory* may have been partly true—and some were certainly exaggerations—but the desired effect was achieved. During the years American was involved in the war, a staggering 400,000 acres of hemp were planted in the United States. (By comparison, America currently plants about 130,000 acres of broccoli.)

Yet the surrender of the Axis powers changed everything once again. In the postwar years, the prohibitions against cannabis went back into force. Government agencies—large and small—went back to cracking down on users and producers alike. In the popular culture of the day, cannabis began to be portrayed as something associated with criminality. Coincidentally, the true research of cannabinoids had just begun in the United States, when cannabidiol (CBD) was first isolated from the molecular structure and researched for its potential benefits.

The Boggs Act of 1952—signed into law by President Harry Truman—mandated that first-time hemp/cannabis-related offenses carry a minimum sentence of two years in jail and a fine of up to $20,000. In a coordinated action, on January 4, 1952—just two months after the Act was passed—five hundred cannabis users were arrested in a coordinated nationwide sweep. (These astonishingly harsh penalties for marijuana possession would remain on the books until 1970!)

In 1969, the academic and counterculture activist Timothy Leary had an important legal case heard by the US Supreme Court. Leary had been arrested for marijuana possession under the Marijuana Tax Act. However, his lawyers argued that the Act was unconstitutional because in situations like Leary's, it could require self-incrimination, which would violate the Fifth Amendment. Leary had been stopped by federal border agents while returning to the US from a trip to Mexico. When asked if he had anything to declare, he did not respond. However, a search of his car revealed marijuana cigarettes and seeds, and he was arrested. Leary's lawyers argued that because marijuana was also illegal in the state of Texas, complying truthfully with the requests of the border agents would be tantamount to incriminating himself under Texas law. Not only did the Supreme Court rule in Leary's favor, but the decision was unanimous.

Leary v. United States had a swift and important fallout. Though the Marijuana Tax Act was now unconstitutional, congress reacted by swiftly passing the Comprehensive Drug Abuse Prevention and Control Act of 1970 and the Controlled Substances Act (which took effect in 1971). These new laws and regulations were the basis for much of the drug control we still have in the United States today. The Comprehensive Drug Abuse Prevention and Control Act was the first to

establish "schedules" for drugs. It required the pharmaceutical industry to be accountable for drug security within these categories and to see that the drugs they produced were correctly categorized into these schedules. The Controlled Substances Act was focused more specifically on preventing the use of illegal drugs by consumers. Among the drugs it targeted was cannabis.

A consequence of these new acts was the establishment of yet another body to enforce them—the Drug Enforcement Administration (or DEA), created in 1973. The DEA was an attempt to consolidate drug enforcement into a single agency, empowered to hunt and arrest violators of federal drug laws of all types.

Even today, the DEA is allowed to investigate any drug it likes—new or old—at any time, and for any reason, should it believe there is a cause to do so. It may choose its own focus and set its own agenda to a great degree. For most of its existence, the DEA has enforced cannabis as a Schedule I drug, meaning that it believes there is no accepted medical use for the drug, and that it is not safe for Americans to use. Despite the fact that in 2019 marijuana is now legal (in one form or another) in 60 percent of all US states, the DEA has still not officially adjusted this status. Many believe that the DEA—like the FBN before it—is loath to admit that a drug may be less dangerous than previously thought, simply because its own budget could be negatively impacted. (Since its creation, the DEA has become one of the most powerful enforcement agencies of any kind in the United States, with a budget now over $2 billion annually.)

Yet as the 1970s drew on, there seemed to be some tentative signs of the pendulum swinging back in the direction of tolerance. Between 1973 and 1977, eleven states decriminalized possession of marijuana (though it remained a federal crime). And the newly elected president, Jimmy Carter, said publicly that he'd like to see marijuana decriminalized. Perhaps most dramatically of all, in October 1977, the Senate Judiciary Committee voted in favor of decriminalizing possession of an ounce or less of cannabis for personal use.

Then the 1980s saw the nation's attitude toward cannabis change once again.

The "Reagan Revolution" saw Republicans take the Executive Branch and a majority in the US Senate. They brought with them a strong antidrug bent and seemed to care little about the potentially positive effects of cannabis. It was as though overnight the budding attitude of permissiveness were driven back entirely. Throughout the 1980s, the DEA enforced a new series of "tough on drugs" policies created by the Reagan administration. These policies called for much harsher sentences for drug-related violations. At the same time, First Lady Nancy Reagan introduced the "Just Say No" campaign and put a friendly face on the war against illegal substances. In the meantime, the new mandatory sentences were enforced for drug offenders. Most of the severe sentences were reserved for drugs like cocaine and heroin, but a few people involved

in transporting or selling very large quantities of cannabis were given very lengthy terms under the harsh new guidelines.

In 1990—near the tail end of the conservative hold on Washington, DC—a new law impacting cannabis and its users was passed, known as the Solomon-Lautenberg Amendment. This law mandated that anyone arrested for drug possession—even for a small amount of cannabis—should have their driver's license suspended for up to six months. The law initially called for states to have their federal highway funds reduced if they refused to comply. However, the law proved unpopular in many places, and the federal government eventually provided states with ways to opt out. Today in 2019, only six states—Alabama, Arkansas, Florida, Mississippi, New Jersey, and Texas—still fully comply with the law and temporarily suspend the licenses of drug offenders; two other states—Michigan and Virginia—partially comply by leaving cannabis off the list of drugs warranting a license suspension. The Solomon-Lautenberg Amendment seemed to be the last shot fired at cannabis by the Regan-era conservatives.

In 1992, the political landscape changed with the election of Bill Clinton to the executive branch and large majorities of Democrats in both the US House and Senate. Suddenly, the US had a president who admitted to having used cannabis personally . . . if somewhat inexpertly. In full, Bill Clinton's famous quote runs: "I've never broken a state law. But when I was in England I experimented with marijuana a time or two, and I didn't like it. I didn't inhale it, and never tried it again." Ever the lawyer, Clinton's legal mind had found a scenario in which he could say that he had tried cannabis—which would certainly connect him with many voters—while still presenting himself as a fully law-abiding citizen.

Clinton may have been the first president to *admit* to using a drug, but he was certainly not the first to partake in mind-altering substances. Presidents back to Washington used laudanum to ease pain. Kennedy was known to have smoked marijuana cigarettes and to have taken amphetamine injections. And even while Clinton was serving as president, a couple of youngsters named George W. Bush and Barack Obama were doing (or had already done) some of their own experimentation involving illegal drugs.

Though many historians have identified the 1990s as the decade when cannabis came onto the cultural, social, and medical "scenes" in an entirely new way, I don't want to give the impression that this change started in those circles with the election of Bill Clinton. In truth, the push to legalize cannabis for legitimate medical use had been fermenting far earlier. What we began to see in the 1990s was the product of many years of hard work by a great number of people—some working together, some on their own—to try and change laws and attitudes about cannabis in order to harness its healing power.

As far back as the middle of the century, advocates had been working to create change

in cannabis perceptions. Though many were dismissed and criticized—or stereotyped in hurtful ways—they kept trying. They grew where they were planted, so to speak, and started organizing to educate the public and alter the dominant ideas and attitudes about cannabis. The work we are able to do today is a direct result of many of their efforts, especially the ones who advocated for the medicinal studies of cannabis.

With that said, let's step back to the pre-Clinton era for a moment and look at how those legalization efforts played out.

In the 1970s and '80s, state legislators began trying to pass laws that would make the medical use of cannabis legal to varying degrees. Slowly but surely, they succeeded. By 1982, over thirty states had some sort of law on the books providing access to "medical marijuana." Some of these states went further, partnering with the federal government to legally supply government-approved cannabis to those who qualified for it. Other states merely passed laws allowing physicians to prescribe cannabis use but failed on the "follow-through" when it came to setting up systems for actually providing that cannabis. Additional states still simply reclassified cannabis to a schedule for drugs with known medicinal properties.

California, however, built on its accomplishments in the '70s and '80s, and then used the '90s to become a true trailblazer.

In 1991 and 1992, laws were passed in San Francisco requiring that law enforcement make medical cannabis its "lowest priority" and allowing physicians to prescribe cannabis to patients with HIV/AIDS. Other cities in California took a page from the San Francisco playbook and began passing their own laws allowing physicians to prescribe cannabis.

Then, in 1996, California voters passed Proposition 215, which legalized not only the use, but the possession and cultivation of cannabis by patients (or their caregivers) with a physician's recommendation. In the same year, voters in Arizona passed a similar law allowing doctors to prescribe cannabis (though it was vetoed in 1998). In the years that followed, a whole host of states—including Washington, Oregon, Alaska, Nevada, Washington, DC, and Maine—passed similar initiatives. Then the floodgates seemed to open, and we have what we have today: a landscape in which thirty-three states (and Washington, DC) have legalized medical cannabis and many more have legalized recreational cannabis (or affirmed that they will no longer prosecute it).

One of the most heartening things about the legalization process has been that we now have years—and in some cases decades—of data to disprove the gloomy forecasts that were made (and sometimes still are made) by opponents of legalization about what an America with increased access to medical cannabis would look like.

While not every opponent of legalization took their position out of spite, insensitivity, or ignorance—and I bear them no personal ill will—I think it is important to point out that they were not correct on some of their most important claims.

Opponents of cannabis claimed that such legalization would result in increased rates of illegal juvenile use and that it would serve as a gateway to harder drugs. They also worried that it would increase crime and lawlessness in general and provide a boost to vice in local communities. Studies now show that, in every case, the opposite has proved true.

Illegal use of cannabis by teens does *not* increase in states where cannabis has been made legal for medical purposes. Rather than serving as a "gateway" and boosting use of other, more serious drugs, studies show that the rate of opioid abuse has *decreased* in states legalizing medical cannabis. And when it comes to crime, studies have found—yep, you guessed it—that violent crime *decreases* in states that legalize medicinal cannabis. Not only this, but since the legalization trend began, violent crime in US states bordering Mexico has also decreased *even if those states have not legalized medical cannabis themselves.* Anyone serious about reducing violence related to drug gangs should be looking hard at the effects of cannabis decriminalization.

Of course, there are still detractors to this day, and they have new claims about the havoc that further legalizing cannabis will surely wreak. Among these arguments is that legalizing cannabis will result in a kind of "THC arms race," as producers try to outdo one another with ever-more potent forms, pushing THC levels to dangerous new heights.

I'm not particularly troubled by these latest objections. I think "superpowerful cannabis" is unlikely to cause large-scale issues. Mostly because of the body's ability to "take what it needs and discard the rest" when it comes to the mobilization of cannabinoids. In other words, you cannot overdose. Furthermore—as you'll see later in this book—cannabis cultivators and growers have responded to the demanding market by manipulating genetics to produce new strains with lower THC and higher CBD content.

So, if that's the journey to how we got here . . . then where is "here"? Where are we right now?

It's a good question, but also a somewhat challenging one to answer because of the constantly changing landscape of cannabis in the United States. There is a chance that even while this book is being printed, another state will pass laws allowing medical marijuana, or another state prosecutor will announce that his or her office will no longer pursue charges related to cannabis. As far as hemp itself is concerned, the passing of the 2018 Farm Bill, allowing for the growth of industrial hemp (or cannabis containing a "less than" percentage of THC), has made the hemp cannabinoid revolution, and CBD, fully possible.

Despite this flux, there are still ways to take stock of what has been accomplished and what still needs to be done.

The crucial year for hemp/cannabis was 2014, when legislators were forced to publicly recognize the differences in cannabinoids, and

more specifically, the plant itself. Though there were some producers of hemp in the United States before this, their ability to navigate a tangled web of legal requirements grew increasingly challenging due to the lack of specifics regarding the allowable content of certain cannabinoids in the plant. The 2018 Farm Bill saw the government "doubling down" on hemp by creating explicit protections for farmers to move hemp products across state lines, to put no limit on the amount of hemp they could grow or possess, and to put no limitations on what their hemp could be used for.

The effect of these prohemp policies has been to give national production a real shot in the arm.

According to a compilation of data from state agriculture reports assembled by Vote Hemp—a national hemp advocacy organization—hemp is now legally grown in twenty-three states. It's still down from that all-time high of 400,000 acres during the Second World War, but over 78,000 acres of hemp were grown in the United States last year—and that number's growing! (The states producing the most hemp are Montana and Colorado; between them, they're responsible for more than half of all US production.) There are over 3,500 licensed growers in the US, and forty-one states either currently allow the cultivation of hemp or have related legislation pending.

There's no telling how fast the industry is going to move from here, but given the explosive growth we've seen thus far, my guess is as fast as it possibly can. An astonishing 511,442

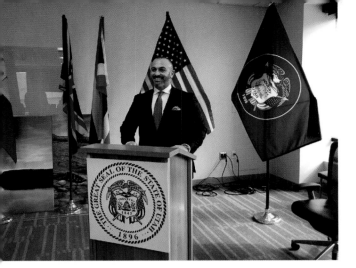

Ryan Lewis speaking to the Utah State Legislature in 2017 on the legalization of hemp.

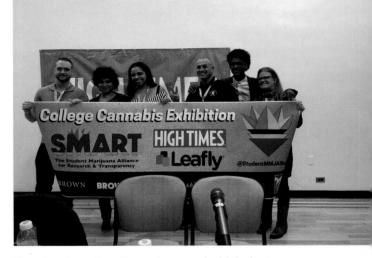

Ryan Lewis on the discussion panel with industry experts at his alma mater, Brown University, for the first cannabis industry job opportunities expo.

acres are licensed to grow hemp in 2019. That's just the licensing, though. How many of those acres will actually be farmed? We'll have to wait until the 2020 state reports to know for sure. It won't be all of them, but it will certainly be far more than last year. Will we be back up to WW II levels soon? My instinct is to say almost certainly yes.

Concurrent with the physical growth of more hemp, our society has seen a growth in the acceptance of cannabis culture. The twentieth-century associations linking cannabis to lawlessness, youth culture, and a particular set of social and political views are slowly receding. States across the country are beginning to expunge criminal convictions related to cannabis. In many cities, the local marijuana dispensary has quickly become as much a part of the neighborhood as the tavern, the hardware store, or the corner grocery. The global legal cannabis industry is now worth tens of billions of dollars.

So I've talked a little about cannabinoids and cannabis in general; however, the rest of this book is going to focus more directly on CBD. At the same time that the presence and availability of cannabinoid THC has grown in this country, so has cannabinoid CBD.

CBD is now legal in every state in the union. (Though it should be noted that some laws exist—for good reason—forbidding CBD products that come from unsafe, unregulated, or untrustworthy sources. More on that later.) Some state governments occasionally attempt to pass their own regional laws regulating CBD, such as requiring a prescription in order for a consumer to access it. However, these laws often fizzle out and are vetoed or overturned.

For CBD to be legal in a state that has not legalized cannabis, a CBD product must not contain more than 0.3 percent of THC. Thus, legal CBD must be made from plants in the United States and must be derived from industrial hemp. This, as you might imagine, causes some confusion and can also create regulatory challenges when a state changes its cannabis laws. Making things even more complicated is the fact that plant strains are not static, and examples exist of hemp crops gradually

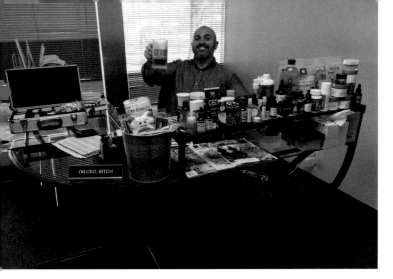

Behind the desk in Colorado Springs where Ryan built his first company into one of the largest vertically integrated hemp CBD operations in the USA.

"evolving" to contain a higher level of THC. This is why having farmers and geneticists in place is vital, so that strains can be bred appropriately and to also gain the desired levels of cannabinoids. Like I said, it's complicated!

The FDA and the DEA have both been involved in the regulation of products containing CBD. Do a quick Internet search, and you can find examples of regulatory actions. However, virtually all cases involve the government investigating a manufacturer—usually for making a fraudulent product or making illegal claims for their marketing. (So far, the DEA has *never* pursued a case against an individual user of CBD or somebody purchasing it for private use.) Sometimes the fight over CBD's legality ends up being a fight over jurisdiction: a law or rule enforced by one agency conflicts with a law or rule from another agency. When this occurs, if both sides refuse to reexamine their interpretation of the rule or law in question, then the matter must be decided by the courts.

To cite an example from this decade, CBD derived from marijuana in the United States remains illegal, falling under an archaic regulation known as the "marihuana extract rule." The suggested 2014 Farm Bill allowed for the growing of hemp—again, a strain of cannabis. When the bill was passed, the DEA challenged this—arguing that hemp was still marijuana and insisting that it should be allowed to pursue growers. However, courts have repeatedly found that the Farm Bill preempts the DEA's mandate to crack down on marijuana . . . at least for the moment.

The legal system's reluctance to decide definitively about the status of CBD leaves open the door to future legal challenges and interpretations. There are scenarios where the government has not yet issued a ruling and probably will not until a legal challenge is mounted. For example, is CBD legal if it is manufactured in the United States but produced from imported hemp with 0.3 percent or less THC content?

The FDA isn't helping much either when it comes to classification and regulation. As discussed in a subsequent section, the FDA is currently classifying CBD as an "Investigational New Drug" for certain conditions and diseases, like epilepsy. That might sound promising, but because of this classification, the FDA cannot concurrently recognize CBD as a dietary supplement. Which is, of course, how a whole lot of people use it.

Competing and conflicting regulatory agencies can place a strain on the ability of CBD product manufacturers to deal squarely and frankly with the public. Currently, the claims that can be made on the packaging of a product containing CBD are few and far between. We're not even allowed to point to the studies and peer-reviewed research that show the benefits CBD can provide for a whole host of conditions. (Fortunately, the laws about the research I can share in a book are very different. That's another reason why I chose to write this!)

Despite these regulatory hurdles, the industry is still growing. People know a good thing when they experience it. The word is out on CBD, and nobody is going to put the toothpaste back in the tube.

CBD use has seen a dramatic rise in the United States. It is happening first in young people, though the other age groups are gradually getting there. According to a 2019 report by the magazine *Consumer Reports*, 40 percent of Americans in their twenties have now tried CBD! The same report found 32 percent of people in their thirties and early forties have tried it, 23 percent of people in their late forties and fifties have, and 15 percent of people aged sixty and older have given it a shot. In total, a little over one quarter of all Americans have now tried CBD, and that number is continuing to rise.

The same report also found that when people do try CBD, they generally regard it as effective. In my opinion, this is as crucial as it should be self-evident; CBD wouldn't be experiencing this remarkable growth if people weren't getting a positive return.

About 75 percent of people who took CBD to treat a specific health issue said that it was at least somewhat effective, and 48 percent said that it was very effective or extremely effective. In addition, a stunning 22 percent said that CBD was so effective that it allowed them to replace a prescription or over-the-counter drug with CBD (with one-third of this 22 percent using it to replace an opioid!).

The same *Consumer Reports* report found that the most common reason people were taking CBD was to relieve stress and anxiety, with 37 percent of users taking it for that purpose. About 24 percent said they took CBD for joint pain. Only 11 percent of respondents said that they had tried CBD "for fun or recreation." (But hey, improving your health with CBD sounds like fun to me! I say more power to them!) As you might imagine, there were differences in who took CBD and why they took it. For example, 32 percent of millennials who used CBD took it for stress, while only 12 percent of baby boomers did. In contrast, 42 percent of baby boomers who used CBD took it for joint pain, while only 15 percent of millennials did. About three-quarters of CBD users take it at least once a day. The vast majority take CBD by ingesting it, either by consuming oil, in pill form, or (the majority) with CBD incorporated into a food. Vaping, topical use, and smoking are also popular. (For that last example, I should clarify that I don't mean smoking marijuana. Multiple manufacturers now make CBD cigarettes, which contain neither tobacco nor cannabis.)

However, the current reports show we've

got a substance that is popular, safe, and effective. So in other words, if this current trend continues, in a few years we could have as many Americans who have tried CBD as those who have a four-year college degree. Yet despite its growing popularity and increasingly widespread use, misconceptions still remain. It is always amusing to me that some of the consumers who can be the biggest evangelists for CBD are still mistaken about some of the basic truths about it.

So where are people picking up their misconceptions?

Multiple studies show that there are three places where most people first learn about CBD: their friends, their family, or the Internet. (It is important to note that physicians—and other healthcare providers—are absent from this list.) Because there are no established government guidelines related to dosing, most of these users are looking to these same sources for information about how much CBD to take, and how to take it.

In my opinion, some of the remaining misconceptions about CBD could be perpetuated by unsavory manufacturers. For example, many users of CBD—especially first-time users—inaccurately believe it is a legal way of obtaining THC, or "getting high." (There are no firm statistics on what percentage of people have made this error. But ask around, and you'll hear many stories of consumers having this experience.) In addition, most consumers also do not know about the source of their CBD. Industry surveys consistently show that about 70 percent of users of CBD don't know how—or from what strain of plant—the CBD in the product they use was extracted.

I believe that, given time, we can correct these misconceptions and help our CBD consumers to be better informed about the products they are purchasing.

I think it is informative to look at how today's consumers are getting their CBD. The ever-changing growth of legal distribution channels can make it challenging to answer the question "Where do people typically obtain their CBD?" The answer is always changing. However, *Consumer Reports* found that in 2019, 27 percent of CBD users said they usually got their CBD from an online source. Other popular answers were at a retail store, or at a dispensary in a state where cannabis is legal. Many people combine sources. For example, they might order CBD online, also buy it in a brick-and-mortar store from time to time, and consume CBD in food on occasion when it is served to them.

One more interesting thing . . .

Increased mainstreaming of CBD and, I believe, increased education are also driving down the number of CBD users who report that they also use cannabis for its CBD properties. A 2015 study by the Center for Behavioral Health Statistics and Quality—a government agency that's part of the Substance Abuse and Mental Health Services Administration—found that 8 percent of Americans used cannabis at least once a month. (This study did not go into whether it was used for

CBD- or THC-related properties.) However, their study from mid-2018 found that only about half of Americans who used CBD regularly also used cannabis at least once a month. I expect these numbers to go down as the public becomes better educated, and as "cannabis culture" and "CBD culture" evolve into their own separate spheres. Many people are fine with just CBD, and that's great!

So, more or less, that's where we are now—and how we got here—when it comes to cannabis and CBD acceptance in the United States. In the next chapter of this book, we're going to look at the *why* of CBD. Why do people use it? Why should they consider using it? What does the latest medical science tell us about what it can do? And where do I think that science is going to take us in the future?

But before I do that, I'd like to conclude this chapter by making it personal. I want to tell you why I think CBD is so important for Americans today, and I want to tell you why it has become my biggest passion.

A NATION AT THE TIPPING POINT FOR POSITIVE CHANGE: MY JOURNEY TO CBD

In my opinion, Americans are sick of being sick. And when it comes to the contemporary

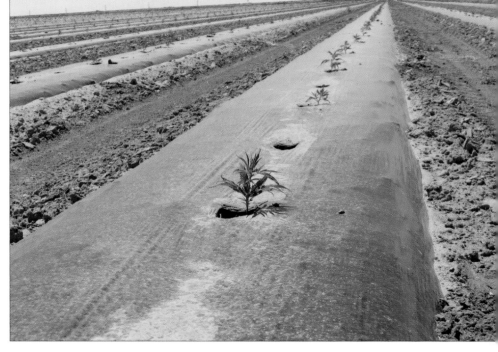

Sproutlings freshly transferred to rich California soil.

offerings in the marketplace that seek to address our medical conditions with chemical pharmaceuticals that carry serious side effects—that can be worse than the condition they claim to cure!—Americans are sick of side effects. So many claims about products related to our health and our bodies turn out to be exaggerated or false. Americans are sick of being disappointed. We would like a better choice—a safe and natural one.

But there are opinions, and then there are facts. And I think the facts speak more loudly than my opinion ever could. It's a fact that our nation is currently in a prescription-drug crisis, and one of the biggest culprits is those used to treat pain.

According to a 2016 report by the CDC, 20.4 percent of US adults now suffer from some degree of chronic pain. (And I should note that some experts have insisted that the real figure is closer to 40 percent.) Moreover, the CDC says that 8 percent of US adults have so-called "high-impact" chronic pain. That's severe and serious pain that significantly limits the ability of the sufferer to engage in normal life activities. Both chronic pain and high-impact chronic pain disproportionately hit the most vulnerable among us—those living in poverty and those without a high school diploma. And chronic pain doesn't usually arrive on its own. It brings along a whole list of partners in crime.

People who suffer from pain are less likely to be active and participate in regular life events. They are more likely to be anxious or depressed. When questioned, they're more likely to say that they have bad health or a poor quality of life. And—vitally—they are more likely to become addicted to opioids.

There may be a number of reasons why Americans are experiencing increased pain. The technology for detecting ailments has improved. There may be less stigma about seeking help for pain. We are also hitting a generational phenomenon as the baby boomers age. Chronic pain tends to become more prevalent with age, as muscles and bones weaken and can no longer provide the kind of support they once could. Elderly Americans are also at a greater risk for the kind of diseases that tend to cause pain.

Enter the opioid crisis. According to the National Institute of Drug Abuse—which is operated by the US Department of Health and Human Services—in 2019, 130 Americans were dying from opioid overdoses *every single day.* These can include deaths from prescription pain relievers, or drugs like heroin and fentanyl. The impact of these deaths tears apart communities, and the government has acknowledged it constitutes it as a massive national emergency. In the hardest-hit areas, local emergency services—from police, fire, and EMTs to emergency department doctors and nurses—find themselves straining to keep up with opioid-related emergencies. Budgets too are strained, as poor rural communities—which can ill afford added expenses under normal circumstances—are pushed to the breaking point by the side effects of opioids. The CDC estimates that $78.5 billion per year is lost in the United States to opioid abuse—in the form of healthcare, lost productivity, and law enforcement expenses. In total, over

Trichomes are tiny hair-like compounds that are often a variety of brilliant colors on cannabis/hemp plants.

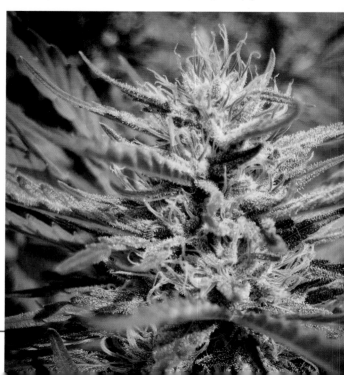

1.5 million Americans are estimated to have a substance abuse disorder connected to prescription opioids.

Entire books have been written regarding what should be done about the opioid crisis, and which forces are to blame for its devastating toll. I'm not going to do that here, but the statistics about prescription opioids in particular make me wonder why doctors would ever recommend something with such potential for misuse as a first line of defense. (According to the National Institute on Drug Abuse, 20 to 30 percent of patients prescribed opioids for pain misuse them. About 5 percent of people prescribed opioids go on to use heroin illegally, and this now accounts for four out of every five heroin users.) Now we see headlines about pharmaceutical companies and executives being investigated for pushing physicians to prescribe a product that they knew to be highly addictive and habit-forming. A product that might take away pain but that would also destroy lives in the process. The government is now moving to address opioid abuse, manufacturers of prescription opioids are being taken to court over false claims, and federal agencies are recommending new approaches to managing pain. Virtually all of these recommendations contain language emphasizing a new path toward nonaddictive strategies. The US Department of Health and Human Services recently announced five major priorities in the fight against opioid addiction, and one of them is "advancing better practices for pain management."

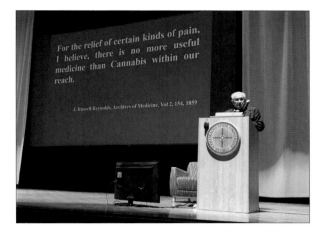

Raphael Mechoulam speaking about the benefits of cannabis in regard to chronic pain.

After the debacle of the opioid crisis, Americans are angry and demanding better solutions. They want supplements that are natural, that won't make them ill with side effects, and that won't become habit-forming (much less create powerful addictions).

And chronic pain is just one example. In the next chapter, we'll look more closely at how CBD shows the potential to make remarkable strides forward as treatment for a whole host of areas—including chronic pain.

The nation is crying out for a solution like CBD.

Think about how frequently we see new studies about the newly discovered negative health consequences of drugs produced by the pharmaceutical industry. Or how frequently we see groups of personal injury lawyers recruiting for a class-action suit against a traditional drug maker.

But sometimes, the simplest solutions are the best solutions.

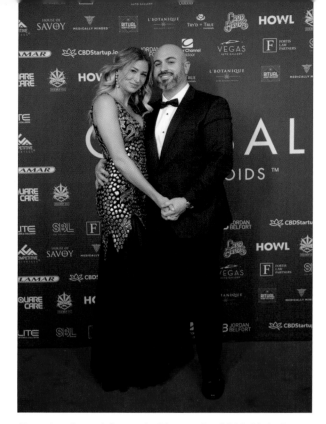

Ryan Lewis and Amanda Rice at the 2019 Global Cannabinoids red carpet holiday event in Las Vegas, NV.

For all the science we'll discuss in this book, CBD is not a complicated mixture of artificial chemicals created in a drug company laboratory. It is an extract from a plant that has been safely used for thousands of years . . . and is only now beginning to be fully understood.

I believe the reason why I'm so personally passionate about CBD is that it connects to the core elements that drive me.

I've always been a person who tried to do two things.

First, I've always been an entrepreneur. Like many of you reading this book, I have tried my best to be a go-getter and to do what I could to grow businesses and create jobs. And I got a pretty early start! Back when I was still an undergraduate at Brown University, I founded a company called Ivy Clean, Inc. It provided reliable cleaning services for dorm rooms and made these services available at a price that even a college student could afford. Ivy Clean was a great way to get my first taste of how to run a company and connect with customers. I launched my own website, took out advertisements, and fielded the calls myself. But I also partnered with preexisting people in the cleaning industry—who already knew the space—to draw on their experience and make sure I could incorporate their best practices from the get-go. While my partnerships might have meant I kept a smaller share of the overall profits, they were worth it because they expanded my reach, allowed me to scale, and improved the overall quality of the product— room cleaning—that I could offer. Ivy Clean was also an exercise in learning how to take advantage of adjacent "low-hanging fruit" in the business space. For example, many students who would pay to have their rooms cleaned would also pay for help with things like packing and unpacking, doing laundry, and other services in that sphere.

It was a great success, but at the end of the day I realized that my calling was not to stay in the cleaning industry for my entire career. Wanting to give back to the school that had given me so much, I donated Ivy Clean to the Brown University Entrepreneurship Program, an organization that I had helped found. I wanted the next generation of students to

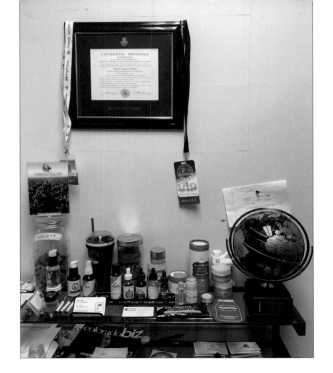

My desk early on in my career, with numerous CBD brands.

have their own chance to run Ivy Clean, so they could get the same real-world business experience that had benefited me, and also to see where they could take it in the future!

The "giving back" of Ivy Clean to the next generation brings me to the other motivating force in my life, namely, the need to make a positive impact and leave the world a better place than how I found it.

I would say that this was instilled in me by all the people in my life who helped guide me and give me values. Most certainly, this list of people includes my friends and family. Another source would be my time in high school in the 1990s at the Marine Military Academy in Texas, the only high school in the United

States that is based solely on the values and traditions of the US Marine Corps. Marines show self-discipline, but they are also willing to do whatever it takes to make the world a better place. It's a special kind of dedication, and I think that more than a little of it rubbed off on me during my time there.

When I graduated college and entered the business world, I remained passionate about retaining a mission-driven aspect to my entrepreneurship. That was what led me to become so intrigued by the promise shown by CBD and to eventually found Global Cannabinoids, Inc., now the nation's top producer, manufacturer, and distributor of American-grown help-derived cannabinoids. We supply the largest companies in the world with the best quality cannabinoids and are the #1 private-label manufacturer of hemp-derived products. We've built a supply chain that stretches across the United States and includes

The first billboard for Entourage Nutritional erected in Colorado in 2017.

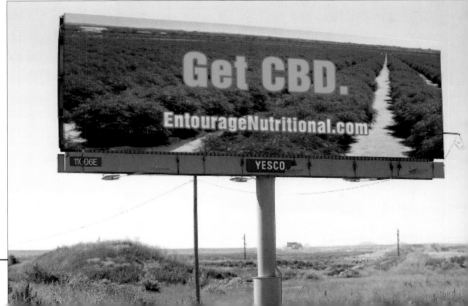

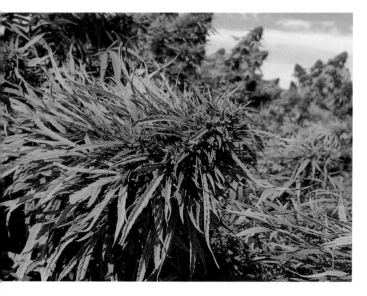

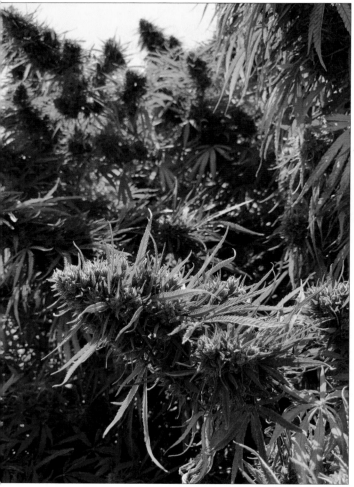

the largest farms, the most advanced extractors, and the best finishers. In my opinion, we provide the best products you can buy!

With all this early success (we've only been around since 2015), you might expect me to be excited—and I am! But I'm not only excited by our success so far . . . I'm excited because we're just getting started!

Every day, I hear about someone whose life has been improved by CBD. It might be somebody with a minor "aches-and-pains" ailment who is now free from pain and able to be more active. It might be someone who uses CBD to simply feel better rested and less anxious. But sometimes it's someone who has dealt with serious chronic pain for years and now, thanks to CBD, feels like they have their life back. Sometimes it's someone who was able to leave behind a serious opioid-based medication for a natural, plant-derived CBD extract. And let me tell you, you don't forget something like that—not when you see it firsthand. These are the big guns! These are the things that really inspire me to keep doing what I do!

I want to make high-quality, safe, and effective CBD accessible to consumers at a reasonable price point, because I've seen the positive impact it can have on people's lives. My work with Global Cannabinoids allows me to pursue my twin passions of being entrepreneurial while making a difference. I genuinely believe that CBD can be one of the main keys to unlocking solutions to the national crisis of opioid addiction and also provide significant relief to the millions of other Americans with health conditions that can be improved or cured with CBD.

Given the exponential growth of CBD thus far—and estimates of how it's going to grow in the future—it's hard to say what the final impact will be. But I'll tell you one thing . . . it's going to be very, very significant.

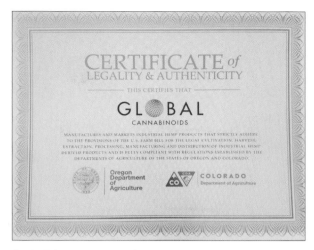

Global Cannabinoids Certificate obtained from Oregon Dept of Ag for cultivation of hemp.

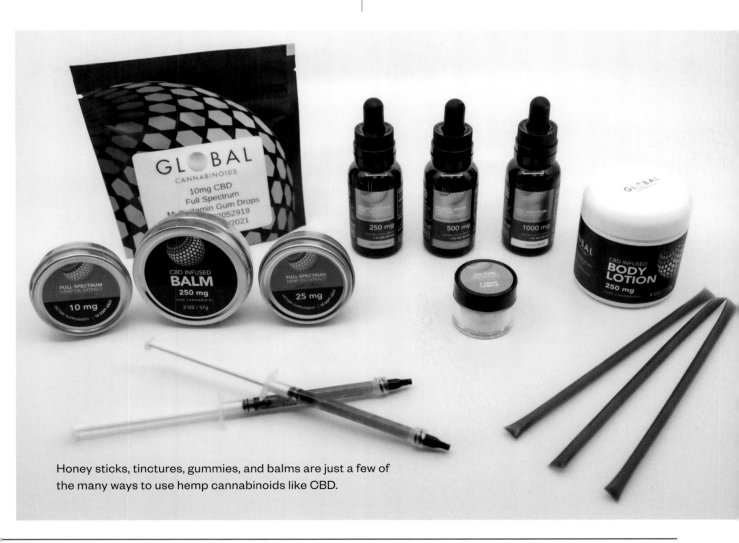

Honey sticks, tinctures, gummies, and balms are just a few of the many ways to use hemp cannabinoids like CBD.

CHAPTER TWO
TREATING HEALTH CONDITIONS WITH CBD

Buds ripe for harvest waving in gentle California breezes.

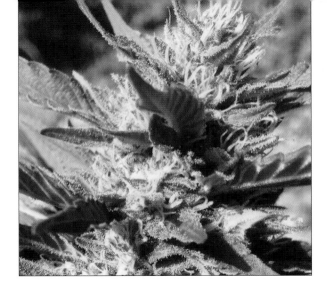

In this chapter, we'll look at the remarkable work being done using CBD to treat specific health conditions. These conditions can run the gamut—from direly serious to merely annoying, and from very common to relatively obscure—but the one thing they have in common is their ability to benefit from being treated with CBD.

This work is not "pure science." That is to say, researchers aren't going into this field because they want to know the effects of CBD with no purpose in mind. We have a purpose in mind: to use CBD to heal people and make their lives better. The results of CBD's effects are increasingly visible in every person who has had a positive response to treatment, who is feeling less pain, and who is living a better and more fulfilling life. Thus, these days, what researchers are generally struggling to understand is the "how" and the "why." Both people with epilepsy and people with chronic pain have benefitted from CBD, for example. That is documented both anecdotally and in peer-reviewed studies. But *why*? What is it about CBD that holds the potential to impact both populations?

As we look at these different diseases and conditions, we'll look at what researchers are finding and what anecdotal evidence tells us. In some areas, scientists are starting to become more confident in their findings. They believe that they are grasping the mechanisms by which CBD works. Yet in other cases, it's still a mystery. Understanding how CBD works is important because that can allow us to understand the applications it may hold for related conditions and symptoms. For example, if CBD helps manage one condition by eliminating inflammation, we know that it may work on related conditions involving that same symptom.

In this chapter, I will cite published, peer-reviewed research to help make my case. CBD-related studies and medical experiments are becoming more and more common, and discoveries sometimes come at breakneck speed. If you are using this book to learn more about a particular medical condition, I encourage you to augment the work cited here with your own research into studies that may have been published after this book was released.

For each condition or disease that we examine, I'll also try to include any available information regarding how CBD can be used to treat it (and/or to prevent it entirely). In some cases, this can involve CBD products available over the counter to consumers now.

At the outset, I want to stress that my advice here **does not replace an appointment with a doctor or other medical professional**.

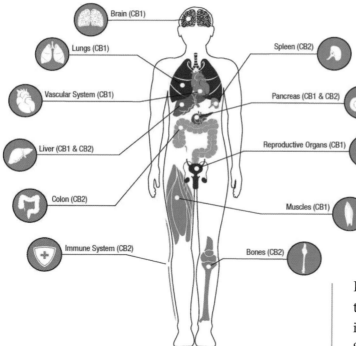

Brain (CB1)

Lungs (CB1)

Vascular System (CB1)

Liver (CB1 & CB2)

Colon (CB2)

Immune System (CB2)

Spleen (CB2)

Pancreas (CB1 & CB2)

Reproductive Organs (CB1)

Muscles (CB1)

Bones (CB2)

CB1 and CB2 receptors are located all over the body, coordinating communications to and from the endocannabinoid system

If you are concerned you may have a serious condition, **seeing a physician should be the first thing you do**. The great thing about CBD is there is no need for a false choice like "using CBD versus using traditional medicine." You can use both. Physicians are increasingly educated about CBD, and can be very receptive to incorporating it into a treatment program. Because CBD's potential for drug interaction is very minimal, it can almost always be used *in addition to*—not instead of—anything your doctor might recommend.

I'm passionate about helping Americans feel better, and part of that means wanting them to do everything they can to make that happen. Now, it may come from CBD, or it may come from CBD used in combination with other treatment options. It's important that we take our health seriously. When facing

a medical condition—even a mild one—it's vital to explore all the information and options available. When consumers do this, I think they'll see what makes CBD such an effective and powerful choice.

EPILEPSY

I wanted to make epilepsy the first condition we examine because it has been uniquely important to the story of CBD in the United States. If there has been one condition that led the scientific community to most-fully embrace the potential of CBD for medical and pharmacological uses, it is probably epilepsy.

Epilepsy is the condition for which the FDA has moved most quickly to greenlight a CBD-based medication. However, as we will see, this move has had both positive and negative consequences for the CBD industry.

A terrifying condition surrounded by many misconceptions and stereotypes, epilepsy can impact anyone, at any stage of life. Some sufferers are born with epilepsy, while others acquire it as a function of age-related deterioration or head trauma. Serious car accidents involving head injuries are a very common cause of epilepsy. It is also a common condition for military veterans who have been injured in explosions. However it is acquired, the symptoms of epilepsy tend to be very similar between patients. Most primarily, they suffer from seizures. Seizures can be so small that an external observer hardly realizes that an epileptic person has had one, or they can be very serious, unmissably violent, involving the entire body. It is challenging for people with epilepsy to maintain normal lives. People with epilepsy whose seizures are not under control can neither drive a car nor participate in activities where they might be injured (or injure others) if they were to suffer a seizure.

Some seizures are not seriously damaging to the epileptic person having them. Other seizures are *very* damaging—the effect on the brain can be like being hit in the head with a hammer. Some sufferers have very occasional seizures, but for others they occur with frustrating regularity.

An astonishing 65 million people worldwide suffer from epilepsy. Some develop it in childhood and "age out" of it as they grow up, but for many less fortunate victims, it stays with them their entire lives. Severe epileptic seizures in children can be barriers to normal mental development. Some forms of epilepsy bring large seizures that can kill suddenly and without warning. And historically—and perhaps most

tragically of all—a large percentage of sufferers have never responded to traditional surgical and pharmacological treatments.

Definitions of epilepsy can vary between countries, or even between states in the US. However, a general rule is that if a person has had more than one seizure, a diagnosis of epilepsy can be appropriate. (Some people use the terms "epilepsy" and "seizure disorder" interchangeably, but others take them to mean two different things—the latter, seizures with an unproven source.)

Though all unnecessary pain represents a tragedy, there is little more upsetting than pain caused to children. Because so many people with epilepsy are born with it, or see it first manifested in childhood, a *very* large community of passionate parents have insisted that the world do more to find ways to fight the disease. (More Americans have epilepsy than have MS, cerebral palsy, muscular dystrophy, and Parkinson's disease *combined*, and yet epilepsy research receives fewer federal research dollars per patient than any of them.)

EEG testing for pediatric patients gives doctors a detailed map and pattern of potentially sporadic waves that the brain makes that may be the cause of seizures.

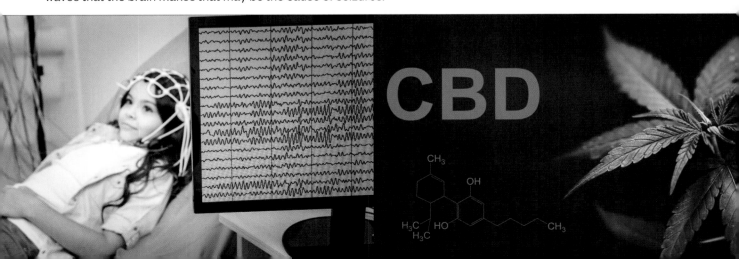

It's important that the fight against epilepsy be being driven by parents, because parents are so wonderful about sharing best practices and tips for what works. Because of this, it was hard to keep CBD's remarkable properties a secret for very long!

The typical journey of a parent of an epileptic child will involve trying a series of medications prescribed by a physician. Physicians will start with the medications that have the greatest chance of success. The parent is told that the first pill prescribed has about a 60 percent chance of controlling their child's seizures. If that pill doesn't work, a second is tried, but parents are cautioned that it has only a 30 percent rate of success. And so on. After the first three or four epilepsy medicines are tried, subsequent medications have a chance of controlling seizures somewhere in the low single digits.

Yet parents of children whose epilepsy is not controlled by the leading drugs—and for whom surgery is not an option—are not ones to give up. They have been historically passionate about exploring the full range of treatment possibilities that yet remain.

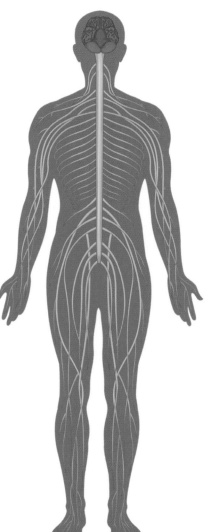

The Nervous System

The first investigation of CBD as a treatment for epilepsy was conducted by the groundbreaking scientist Dr. Raphael Mechoulam (about whom I'll write more in a later chapter) in 1980. Long suspecting that CBD could be useful for epileptics, he started with animal models and found good results and then conducted the first human trial in Brazil. The trial involved giving half of a group of epileptics who suffered seizures 200–300mg of CBD daily for 4.5 months—in addition to their regular anti-seizure medications—and the other half a placebo. About 50 percent of the test subjects given CBD reported no seizures at all, and most of the rest reported at least some improvement in reducing their frequency of seizures. Only about 12 percent given the CBD saw no impact at all on their seizures.

Unbelievably, when the results of this study were published, there was little-to-no notice in the medical and scientific community. This may have been because of prejudice against a substance derived from cannabis. It may have been that Dr. Mechoulam was the only one working on CBD as a treatment for seizures. But looking back today, it seems astonishing—and downright upsetting—that the potential positive impacts for CBD on epileptics then lay dormant *for another thirty years!*

In the mid-2010s, enough parents (and physicians) had tracked down the 1980 experiment that new studies began to be run. Those studies continue today, and the findings have been remarkable . . . yet it was still a fight! Most epilepsy researchers and nonprofits rely on substantial government funding to make progress—funding that politicians can theoretically decide not to renew. Without indulging in political stereotypes, many researchers have hesitated to delve into CBD—and many nonprofits have hesitated to officially endorse its salutary properties on their websites—because they're concerned that politicians (or their constituents) will misunderstand it as "recommending marijuana for children." Which, of course, could not be further from the truth.

One of the current challenges with CBD and epilepsy is that, while it clearly works, researchers are still not exactly sure why. Not every person with epilepsy (or a seizure disorder) experiences a positive result with CBD, but many do. This may be because of genetic factors, or because of the kind of epilepsy that the patient has. Some scientists think the key to unlocking CBD and epilepsy may lie in the molecular targets of CBD. There are sixty-five candidates, but researchers now believe that only fifteen of them are likely to be the one(s) that matter when it comes to epilepsy. Some researchers are now focusing on receptors involved in regulating transmissions between synapses in the brain; these receptors send molecules between neurons. Because seizures can happen when this exchange of molecules becomes exaggerated or hyperactive, it is thought that CBD may block the receptors that allow the exchange of these molecules.

Another theory is that CBD helps control epilepsy because it impacts adenosine—an anticonvulsant occurring naturally in the body. Many researchers have pointed out that it would be intuitive that CBD stops seizures because it boosts adenosine, but there's no scientific proof yet. Overwhelmingly, the "proof" scientists have is simply that CBD tends to control seizures without causing side effects.

A 2017 study in children with a form of epilepsy called Dravet Syndrome—and whose seizures had not been controlled by other medicines—found that CBD was proven effective at reducing convulsive seizures. Other studies have found that CBD was effective in reducing seizures in children with another variety of epilepsy called Lennox-Gastaut Syndrome. Then last year, an FDA panel finally approved a CBD-based medicine called Epidiolex to treat certain epilepsies in children. For many advocates of CBD, this was a watershed moment and a vindication.

Yet on the day Epidiolex was made legal, FDA Commissioner Scott Gottlieb released a statement that read in part:

> Controlled clinical trials testing the safety and
> efficacy of a drug, along with careful review

through the FDA's drug approval process, is the most appropriate way to bring marijuana-derived treatments to patients. Because of the adequate and well-controlled clinical studies that supported this approval, prescribers can have confidence in the drug's uniform strength and consistent delivery that support appropriate dosing needed for treating patients with these complex and serious epilepsy syndromes. We'll continue to support rigorous scientific research on the potential medical uses of marijuana-derived products and work with product developers who are interested in bringing patients safe and effective, high quality products. But, at the same time, we are prepared to take action when we see the illegal marketing of CBD-containing products with serious, unproven medical claims. Marketing unapproved products, with uncertain dosages and formulations can keep patients from accessing appropriate, recognized therapies to treat serious and even fatal diseases.

The FDA giveth, and the FDA taketh away! That was how many of us on the leading edge of CBD felt. Though it might have seemed like an innocuous bit of common sense, Commissioner Gottlieb's decision to make remarks about health claims created serious disappointments in CBD circles. It had been hoped that the definitive demonstration of CBDs effectiveness and safety for the FDA might have led to a more permissive stance on making true statements about the product. Yet here, the commissioner seemed to be saying that only CBD products that had been through extensive double-blind testing—Epidiolex was tested on 516 patients, for example—would be able to talk about the positive things that we've proved, time and again, that CBD can do. The FDA seemed to be saying, "Yes, it looks like CBD can have a positive impact on epilepsy, but you're only allowed to talk about it if your drug has gone through the 'FDA ringer' and come out again."

Even though the FDA used the announcement regarding Epidiolex to try to control who would be able to share the research results linked to CBD (and in what contexts), the approval of the drug was still a milestone. The FDA approval helped many parents of epileptic children feel more comfortable making the choice to try CBD as an easily accessible form of medication. No longer did it seem pseudoscientific or associated with recreational marijuana use. And for the rest of us in the CBD community? Well, we were proven right once again. The overall profile of CBD was raised and made more legitimate. The hope now is that, as continued research shows more and more of what CBD can do, the FDA will finally relax its position on the claims manufacturers can make. (Can you imagine if the FDA did not allow manufacturers of aspirin to say their product helped to reduce fever and relieve pain? That's a bit of what it feels like for us right now.)

Because of its groundbreaking status as being FDA-approved to treat epilepsy, I think it's safe to say that CBD knowledge and acceptance in the epilepsy community will continue to grow—and I believe that people

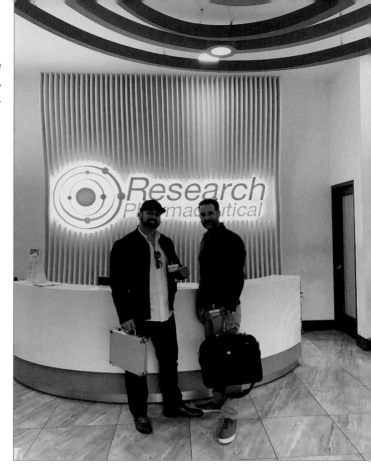

with children who have benefited from CBD for their epilepsy can become some of our most powerful supporters. The major epilepsy nonprofits that people turn to after a diagnosis—like the Epilepsy Foundation and CURE Epilepsy—are talking about it and sharing resources on their websites. Parents are sharing information in online groups and newsletters. And physicians who treat epilepsy are talking to one another about this new treatment option.

I also think it is only a matter of time before folks in the epilepsy community start to wonder if this newly approved medicine could also help other conditions that they or their loved ones have. Looking forward, I predict that some of CBD's strongest change agents are going to emerge from the epilepsy world.

Let me finish up on the subject by answering some questions people generally have at this point: Can taking CBD regularly prevent epilepsy from occurring prophylactically? Currently, there's no evidence for or against that. We just don't know. Someone for whom epilepsy "runs in the family" might certainly want to take any step that might prevent it from occurring. Hopefully, future research will tell us if CBD could ward off developing epilepsy that is inherited.

What about epilepsy due to traumatic brain injury? As discussed in a subsequent section on CBD and injury (p. 65), at least one study has found that using CBD may reduce the chance of death when someone suffers a TBI. So far, no study has explored whether CBD users also had a lower chance of developing epilepsy after a TBI. However, it stands to reason that if CBD use makes the brain less susceptible to fatal injury, it might also help protect it from diseases like epilepsy. Hopefully, more research will soon help us to answer this question.

If you have a recent diagnosis of epilepsy, you should know that there are many treatments that have been shown to work. Your treatment should always be coordinated through a medical professional. Don't try to treat seizures yourself with over-the-counter CBD products as a first line of defense. That said, don't be surprised if your physician recommends a treatment involving CBD. And if you're one of the thousands of epileptics for whom "nothing has worked," I strongly advise you to circle back with your healthcare provider to see if a CBD-based treatment might be right for you.

CHRONIC PAIN

Chronic pain is a condition that impacts millions of Americans. I wrote a bit about chronic pain in the last chapter, as I believe it makes such a compelling case for the importance of treatment options like CBD. I want to circle back to it here because it's a rich topic with many unique aspects to explore. One of these is its history as a central driver for studies that examine the relationship between cannabinoids and medical treatment.

It is almost impossible to discuss CBD's use to treat chronic pain without looking at the history of cannabis, as well. Studies have shown for decades that cannabis use—such as smoking marijuana—is effective in reducing many different types of pain, be it neural or muscular. This verified effect is one of the more powerful forces that has gradually given birth to the "medical marijuana" movement. However, the THC contained in marijuana does produce a "high" that may not be appropriate for every pain patient, as some people may be predisposed to THC addiction. Others may need medication that will not impair their ability to work or drive a car. Others still may simply not like the effects of THC.

But luckily for us, new research is showing that a substantial portion of cannabis's

pain-killing effects may not be related to THC, but rather to CBD.

The earliest studies on CBD and pain simply sought to answer the question "Does CBD alleviate pain at all?" Some believed that the claims of CBD's positive impact on pain were merely psychosomatic effects, or came from people who had confused CBD with THC.

In 2003, an important study was conducted when a group of British researchers recruited volunteers from pain relief clinics and solicited referrals from physicians for patients who suffered from chronic pain. The study was titled "Initial experiences with medicinal extracts of cannabis for chronic pain: Results from 34 'N of 1' studies" and published in the journal *Anaesthesia* in 2004. All patients studied were at least eighteen years of age and had been generally unresponsive to other

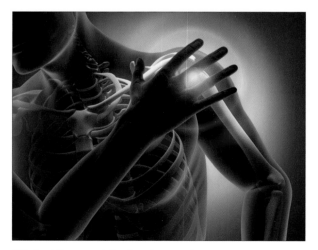

Clinical Research is showing us that compounds like CBD reduce inflammation in the body by activating the endocannabinoid system.

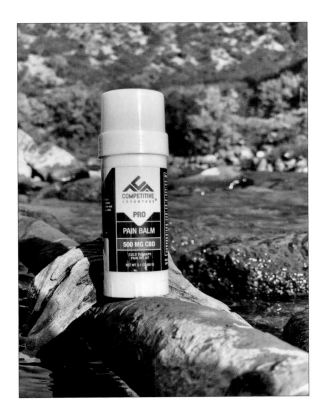

methods of addressing their chronic pain. The patients were first given an oral spray that combined THC and CBD—and observed for responses and side effects—and then given a second spray that contained *either* THC or CBD, but not both (while a control group was given a placebo). The patients filled out a general health questionnaire to note if the spray might be impacting their sleep or other aspects of their lives. (The researchers found that side effects were mild and included drowsiness and dry mouth—similar to the side effects reported by the placebo group.) The subjects were also questioned about their chronic pain.

When it came to pain control, the researchers reported that overall, "Extracts which contained THC proved most effective in symptom control" but also noted that CBD alone was still often effective for many patients. (It is hard, now, to visualize how revolutionary this finding must have been in 2003—a time when many expected that CBD would, in effect, do nothing.) In fact, the researchers reported that some patients also found CBD as effective as the original medication. No patient found the placebo as effective as the original medication. This blew the researchers' minds! In some cases, CBD *was as effective as THC* when it came to controlling pain. The researchers called for additional studies into the ability of both THC and CBD to eliminate chronic pain.

Subsequent studies and laboratory research have allowed physicians to better understand what is going on with pain patients who take CBD. The findings concluded that CBD does not relieve pain by producing a narcotic effect, but rather by reducing inflammation and inhibiting other pain-causing elements in the nervous system. Some studies have also found that CBD can stop the body from absorbing anandamide, a natural compound associated with reducing pain. More—and longer—anandamide presence may mean patients naturally experience less pain.

More studies are still needed for isolating exactly how it works, but the important thing at the moment is researchers are finding that it *does* indeed work.

CBD helps with chronic pain, period.

Sometimes, researchers are even surprised by the *ways* in which CBD finds a way to inhibit pain. For example, one study that tested the benefits of CBD on patients with multiple sclerosis (MS) concluded that CBD reduced spasticity in these patients. But, crucially, this reduction in spasticity led to a reduction in pain. (Limbs that were less spastic felt better.) A different study from 2012 testing the impact of CBD on glycine receptors found that CBD reduces inflammation and that this action reduced chronic pain.

Another added benefit of using CBD to treat chronic pain is that patients do not seem to develop a tolerance to CBD. With many pain treatments—from THC to opioids—patients adjust to the medicine and are forced to increase their dosage to achieve the same effects. This can carry increased dependence and risks of future health problems. CBD, on the other hand, does not appear to have this problem. Patients have not shown signs of building up a tolerance, and doses have not needed to be continuously adjusted. Because the FDA does not currently regulate or recommend dosing for CBD, this has an added benefit for users who

will have to work to find the dosage that works best for them.

Even though the mechanisms are still being understood—and even though CBD may attack pain on a variety of unique fronts for each user—the ability to control pain has been an incredible revelation for early users of CBD.

The 2018 study "A Cross-Sectional Study of Cannabidiol Users" by Jamie Corroon and Joy A. Philips, published in the journal *Cannabis and Cannabinoid Research*, found that chronic pain is now *the most common reason* that many individuals take CBD. Nearly 36 percent of respondents who said they took CBD for chronic pain (or another medical condition) said that it treated their condition "very well by itself," meaning that no other medicines were necessary for regulating the pain. Like others before them, the researchers in this study also concluded that the reduction in chronic pain people were experiencing

Ryan Lewis with champion of cannabis, Raphael Mechoulam

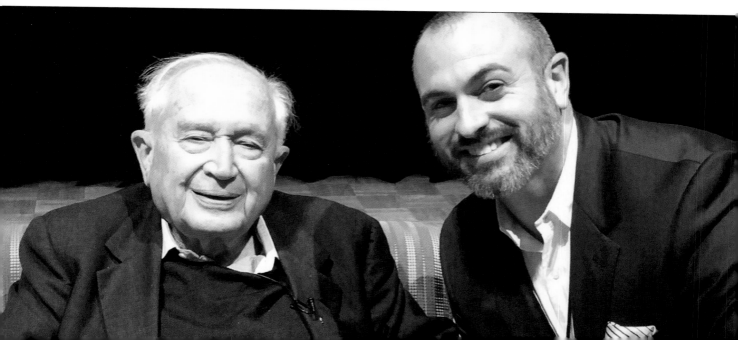

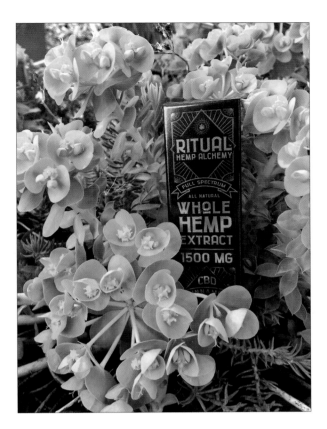

through using CBD was probably primarily related to inflammation. As the study put it:

> The most common medical condition for which CBD was reportedly used was pain. In preclinical studies, CBD-based analgesia is associated with potent immune-modulatory, anti-inflammatory, and antioxidant activity. CBD acts as an agonist for a wide variety of cell-surface receptors including adenosine A2A, 5-HT1A, TRPV1, α7nAch, α3 glycine receptors, and the peroxisome proliferator-activated receptor gamma (PPAR-γ) nuclear receptor. These receptors are all associated with anti-inflammatory activity. Consistent with the efficacy reported by survey respondents, CBD has been shown to reduce inflammatory cytokines in murine models of inflammatory disease and chronic and acute pain.
>
> The endocannabinoid system may also play a role in CBD-mediated analgesia. CBD inhibits enzymes (i.e., fatty acid amide hydrolase and monoacylglycerol lipase) that degrade endocannabinoids. This inhibition is associated with increased endocannabinoid levels, analgesia, and opioid-sparing effects in preclinical models of pain.

In other words, people are using CBD for pain because they find it effective. Based on how CBD interacts with the body, the researchers found scientific underpinnings for this effectiveness.

Another study published last year in *The Journal of Pain Research*, titled "Pharmacotherapeutic considerations for use of cannabinoids to relieve pain in patients with malignant diseases," found through a series of double-blind tests that cannabinoids were effective in reducing pain in patients with serious conditions about 80 percent of the time. Not all of the pain reductions were enormous, but pain reduction is pain reduction.

A remarkable thing is that CBD seems to be effective for almost every *type* of pain. The pain can come from an injury or a disease, or it can be the side effect of a medical treatment. Whatever the origin of the pain, CBD treats it effectively without risk of addiction. Several countries outside of the United States have already begun to use this research for greenlighting the approval of CBD explicitly for the treatment of pain. However, in the United States, the FDA has yet to allow manufacturers to point out CBD's observable pain-killing properties.

But what about conditions *adjacent* to pain, like anxiety, depression, and sleeplessness?

While not the same as pain precisely, these conditions cause extreme discomfort and suffering in millions of people. We'll look at each of these later in this chapter, but as it happens, the new research is also showing improvements in these areas, as well. The fact that CBD is effective at treating all of these is very important because, for many sufferers, the conditions are interlinked. It's not true in every case, but some people are anxious, and depressed, and have trouble sleeping—all at the same time—because they are suffering from a multitude of issues including chronic pain. While the drug industry has produced medications for treating these conditions individually, they've had varying degrees of success. Moreover, many of the most commonly prescribed treatments are potentially addictive and/or carry significant side effects.

CBD, on the other hand, has been proven effective at addressing these interlinked conditions connected to pain with no serious side effects for users. Some researchers believe that it is CBD's ability to positively impact serotonin receptors that accounts for its ability to so seamlessly and safely regulate mood and sleep, in addition to pain.

Despite FDA reluctance thus far, there is growing evidence that CBD's ability to fight pain may be the next thing to move the needle when it comes to new legislation.

In late 2019, the National Institutes of Health (NIH) announced approval of a multi-million-dollar grant to research the effects of cannabinoids for pain relief. The government was specific that these research funds will *not* cover research into THC, only CBD. In a rare admission that they've been behind the eight ball when it comes to CBD, the announcement of the new research funds came with a quote from the deputy director of the National Center for Complementary and Integrative Health—part of the NIH—David Shurtleff, in which he admitted: "The science is lagging behind the public use and interest [when it comes to CBD]. We're doing our best to catch up here. These new projects will investigate substances from cannabis that don't have THC's disadvantages, looking at their basic biological activity and their potential mechanisms of action as pain relievers." The money for this project from the NIH will fund several pain-related studies at colleges and universities across the country.

In addition to catching up with CBD's adoption into our culture, there's also evidence that the NIH's focus on CBD is related to the government's similarly belated efforts to do something about the opioid crisis. The director of the NCCIH, Helene Langevin, said as much in the same announcement: "The treatment of chronic pain has relied heavily on opioids, despite their potential for addiction and overdose and the fact that they often don't work well when used on a long-term basis. There's an urgent need for more effective and safer options."

You can say that again!

It's heartening to see that the government is moving ahead with funding CBD research

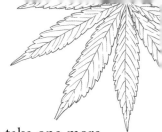

in this area. Again, we need more research, not less. We have nothing to hide about this substance and want the government to serve as an ally when it comes to getting the word out about the benefits of CBD—especially when it comes to those who would be able to use it for reducing serious pain. It's too early to know what the impact of these NIH-funded studies will be on the industry, but my experience tells me that the findings will show that CBD does help to fight pain, and that it does so through an entirely different mechanism from opioids or THC.

If you personally suffer from pain that has not been eliminated by other treatments, I strongly encourage you to give CBD a try. If you don't want to stop any other pain treatments you may already be taking, you probably won't have to. Talk to your physician managing your pain. CBD can almost always be added to an existing pain control regimen without interfering with the original treatment.

I should add that if you're feeling pain for the first time and don't know the cause, you can take some CBD for it if you'd like, but also be sure to see your physician. In some cases, pain can be our body's way of telling us that we need to take medical action.

People who have been living with chronic pain have traveled a long, difficult journey. There's no two ways about it. I've met enough of them personally to know how much they suffer and how brave they have to be. If you are someone who falls into this category, I

hope that you'll be willing to take one more step in this hard journey and try CBD . . . you may find that it's the best one you've taken yet!

ANXIETY

Anxiety is an area in which cannabinoids of all types—but CBD in particular—are showing real potential to provide strong benefits for consumers. Users of cannabis have known for centuries—millennia, according to some—of the power of cannabinoids to counteract anxiety. (While a small percentage of cannabis users can report feeling panic the first time they try the substance, vastly more discover that it has the ability to reduce their anxiety.) As noted above, the ability of CBD to reduce anxiety seems to be connected to its ability to reduce connected problems like pain, depression, sleeplessness, and inflammation. While its mechanisms are still being studied, any tool for reducing anxiety is sure to be welcomed by an increasingly anxious nation.

According to the Anxiety and Depression Association of America (ADAA), all anxiety disorders, combined, now constitute the most common form of mental illness in the United States, with over 18 percent of the total population suffering from them. And as with so many other medical conditions, the numbers will only continue to rise. In 2018, an American Psychiatric Association (APA) survey found that almost 40 percent of Americans reported being *more* anxious than they had been during the same time in the previous year. About the same number of respondents said they were equally anxious, and only 19 percent said they were feeling less anxious.

Some people seem to be more naturally anxious than others: those who simply have a baseline predisposition toward anxiety and nervousness. However, factors like stress, brain chemistry, and life events can all impact how and why we feel anxious.

The 2018 APA study also found that personal and family safety, personal health, and finances were the biggest anxiety triggers for Americans. A whopping 68 percent of Americans surveyed said that keeping themselves and their families safe and/or their own personal health were causes of anxiety in their lives. About 58 percent of Americans said that "politics" was something that could make them feel anxious, and 48 percent said that finances, relationships with friends, family members, or work colleagues cause them to feel anxious. In addition to triggers, the APA research concluded that Americans overwhelmingly regard anxiety as a negative physical state with real consequences. About 86 percent of respondents agreed that anxiety

Sunset on the hemp fields in Colorado.

had a negative impact on a person's physical health and wellness.

Globally, there is the sense that anxiety may be just as high as—or higher than—what we see in the United States . . . yet chronically underdiagnosed. For example, a large study published in *JAMA Psychiatry* in 2017 found that when it came to diagnosis of Generalized Anxiety Disorder, or GAD (which is only one form of anxiety that can be diagnosed), 5 percent of residents of high-income countries had GAD, 2.8 percent of residents of middle-income countries had GAD, but only 1.6 percent of residents of poor countries had GAD. Scientists are still trying to make sense of these numbers. Some think that in middle- and low-income countries, anxiety is more likely to be diagnosed as another condition, like depression. Another fact complicating the matter is that people tend to experience less anxiety as they age. (For example, the 2017 study "Predictors of remission from generalized anxiety disorder and major depressive disorder" published in the *Journal of Affective Disorders* found that a significant predictor of experiencing GAD remission is simply reaching old age.)

There are a number of factors at play when it comes to understanding anxiety globally, and clearly there's more research to be done.

Whatever the cause and whatever the prevalence, those suffering from anxiety want relief! According to the ADAA, over one-third of all Americans suffering from anxiety seek some form of medical or professional treatment.

The last century has seen a large uptick in the development of traditional pharmaceutical medications to treat anxiety. Most of these have involved benzodiazepines—which are better known by their brand names like Xanax and Klonopin. While often effective, these drugs also offer a high potential for abuse, misuse, and dependency. They can be dangerous when someone takes more than the prescribed amount. Yet despite these drawbacks, they remain widely prescribed and very popular.

But why not CBD? Why not a substance that is safe, that produces no "high," and that preexisting evidence suggests is quite effective? The mainstream scientific community is now beginning to ask these same questions, and their experiments and studies tend to confirm what proponents of cannabinoids already know.

In 2010, the study "Neural basis of anxiolytic effects of cannabidiol (CBD) in generalized social anxiety disorder: a preliminary report" published in the *Journal of Psychopharmacology* found that CBD was very effective in treating patients with generalized social anxiety disorder. The study involved a double-blind procedure in which subjects were given either 400mg of CBD or a placebo and then had physiological factors for anxiety measured. Then, in a second session, the participants were switched: those who had received a placebo now received CBD, and so on. The researchers found that while the subjects receiving the placebo showed no reduction in anxiety, those taking CBD showed "significantly decreased" anxiety.

A 2014 study titled "Antidepressant-like and anxiolytic-like effects of cannabidiol: a chemical compound of Cannabis sativa" published in *CNS and Neurological Disorders* found that CBD had both antianxiety and antidepressant effects. A 2015 analysis "Cannabidiol as a Potential Treatment for Anxiety Disorders" published in the journal *Neurotherapeutics* found that CBD could be an effective treatment for many specific subtypes of anxiety. The analysis concluded that all evidence strongly supports CBD as an effective treatment.

In 2016, *The Permanente Journal* published "Effectiveness of Cannabidiol Oil for Pediatric Anxiety and Insomnia as Part of Posttraumatic Stress Disorder: A Case Report." This piece chronicled CBD's effective role in treating anxiety brought on by PTSD and manifesting itself in the form of sleeplessness. The author found that CBD proved effective in relieving the anxiety that was causing the sleeplessness.

And a study published in early 2019 in the *Brazilian Journal of Psychiatry* titled "Cannabidiol presents an inverted U-shaped dose-response curve in a simulated public speaking test" produced some of the most interesting and compelling results of all. This study found that CBD was effective in combating anxiety and that using CBD to decrease

anxiety worked even though "the molecular and neural mechanisms involved in the anxiolytic effects of CBD are incompletely understood." This article used research taken from subjects who were suffering from anxiety and had been administered one 300mg dose of CBD (or a placebo) and then asked to give a speech about public transportation that was recorded on camera, and with a monitor displaying a live image of the speaker in front of them. (This was designed to heighten anxiety, as public speaking is a major source of fear and anxiousness for many people.) At various points during the speech, the participant was interrupted to have their vital signs taken for any indicators of stress. A follow-up study tried the same thing, but with 600mg. In both studies, researchers had found that "treatment [with CBD] was associated with significant reductions in anxiety, cognitive impairment, and distress during the speech, as well as with reduced arousal during the anticipatory phase." That is to say, people who took just one dose of CBD were less nervous during their speeches, and also in the time directly before speaking. The researchers also found that the anxiety-reducing effects of CBD were lessened if they gave the participants too little, and also if they administered too much. This is important because it establishes that

1. CBD definitely has a positive impact on reducing anxiety; and

2. Dosing is real and important, and increasing the amount of CBD administered is not always proportionate to increasing the degree to which their anxiety is relieved.

The researchers concluded, rightly, that more work needed to be done when it comes to formulating the best CBD doses to combat anxiety.

In both animals and humans, CBD has been repeatedly shown to exhibit powerful antianxiety effects. This may be connected to CBD's anti-inflammatory function, or it may occur through an entirely different chemical mechanism. This is something scientists are still studying. But however it works, folks are coming into agreement that something good is happening. Even the notoriously cautious Mayo Clinic, in a 2019 post on its blog on the topic, somewhat grudgingly noted that using CBD to treat anxiety is "associated with some symptom improvement." The same blog points to a January 2019 study that found CBD improved the anxiety of 57 out of 72 participants in a trial. That's 79 percent!

As anybody who has suffered from anxiety can tell you, it is a complicated medical condition. Its symptoms can result in public "flare-ups" that are very noticeable—like panic attacks or anxiety attacks—but can also be a burden borne silently by the sufferer. There still remains a substantial stigma surrounding anxiety, too. Some people feel that because anxiety isn't something you can "see"—like a broken bone or a flu bug—it somehow isn't real. But again, people who suffer from anxiety can tell you its all too real, and that it can make their lives incredibly difficult.

On the upside, anxiety is something that can be attacked from many different directions. I hope that for people with anxiety, CBD feels like just one more "weapon in their arsenal." Talk therapy, meditation, exercise, deep breathing, mindfulness, and medications are useful in treating anxiety and can be used in combination.

In the CBD community, we've come to the conclusion that people taking CBD for anxiety find there's no one "right way" when it comes to technique and dosing. Some with anxiety find that taking CBD on a regular schedule—once in the morning and once in the evening, for example—can help keep their symptoms under control throughout the day. Others find that it can be helpful to take CBD during a flare-up of anxiety, using a "fast delivery" method, such as dissolving a tincture under the tongue or inhaling vaporized CBD (more on these delivery methods in a subsequent chapter). Sudden panic attacks can make people with anxiety feel like they're suddenly going to pass out or have a creeping sense of doom. For these folks, the idea of a fast-acting CBD delivery method is especially cheering and could greatly reduce human suffering. Each person with anxiety should feel comfortable experimenting with CBD as a treatment to find the application that works best for them, while also working with their physician and/or psychiatrist.

SKIN CARE AND PERSONAL APPEARANCE

Skin health can be an important indicator of our overall well-being. Allergic reaction, irritation, stress, and disease can all make themselves known through skin irritation. On top of this, our skin—especially the skin on our faces—is the most visible part of our bodies. It's the one we use to communicate emotions, give social cues, and show our reactions. As any teenager can tell you, people who suffer from disruptions on their skin, like acne, often feel anxious and self-conscious about their appearance. This, in turn, can lead them to become more introverted and less sure of themselves. You don't have to take my word for it; there's a reason Americans spent an astounding $135 billion on skincare products in 2018!

Yet skin is unique. Skin tones are unique. And most certainly, the varying forms of skin conditions are unique, as well. Try as it may, the skincare industry has yet to craft a "magic bullet" that provides perfect relief for the most common issues.

But hold on a second . . . it is now starting to look like that magic bullet might just be CBD.

To the naked eye, our skin is a telltale indicator of so many health issues our bodies are processing because *it shows inflammation* (or

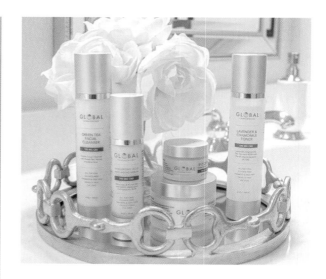

becomes inflamed). The most common sort of skin inflammation is acne. At any given moment, about 10 percent of the population has some form of acne. CBD may directly help control acne because of its tendency to reduce inflammation. A lack of endocannabinoids may be another reason for outbreaks in the skin. While the precise role in skin is being understood, conditions like acne, inflammation, and eczema stand to be corrected by CBD according to this science.

In addition to acne and inflammation, CBD may help with overall skin health and appearance—reducing visible inflammations and reactions. CBD is also a very safe choice. The skincare industry offers everything from chemical peels to Botox injections (a literal toxin!) to prescription medications that can have serious side effects. CBD offers to potentially provide benefits that will keep our skin looking and feeling healthy in a number of ways while eliminating the need for riskier alternatives.

CBD also shows that it can eliminate the excessive activation of the immune system in allergic reactions. Because of this, CBD treatments may hold the promise of treating skin allergies and immune-related diseases of the skin.

Because hair follicles are a part of our skin, I'll note that there is even reason to believe that CBD may hold the key to new and more effective treatments for balding and/or eliminating unwanted hair. Hair follicles can continue to grow hairs over the course of our entire lives. However, when hair follicle CB1 receptors are activated, the cell division stops and the follicle stops growing. Because CB1 is involved—and because of the powerful interaction of CBD and CB1—it is likely that one day soon we will understand the potential of CBD to *prolong* hair growing by hair follicles. (It is also possible that this will, one day, allow us to reverse engineer the process and use the same mechanism to eliminate unwanted hair safely and naturally.)

CBD helps our skin look and feel better on a number of fronts, and another key to understanding how and why is also connected to its impact on pain, anxiety, and even seizures. The key word is *inflammation*. The skin protects our body from environmental dangers but is also an active organ. Without it, life as we know it would not be possible. Our outer layer of skin is always hard at work, healing and repairing itself.

The outermost layer of our skin is called the epidermis, which is formed by layers of epithelial cells called keratinocytes. The epidermis is designed to protect against UV radiation, microbes, and contaminants and chemicals that might be found in the environment.

The next layer of our skin is where we find hair follicles, sebaceous glands, and sweat glands. This second layer is considered very active, as our follicles are always expending energy growing new hair. Our sebaceous glands are constantly supplying oily sebum up to the layer of skin above it. Our sweat glands are always working to regulate the body's temperature. This layer of skin also produces steroids and Vitamin D to help with the skin's immune defense. (Our skin really has its own little immune system that is ever at work trying to keep us safe from bacteria and

Organic ingredients like Calendula and Comfrey are often combined with whole hemp to create effective creams and salves.

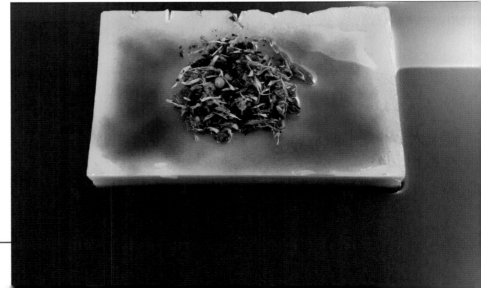

viruses. Immune cells are alive inside our skin, and they know they have work to do whenever we come into contact with a threat. Our skin's immune system works tremendously hard to keep us safe.)

Beneath those upper layers of skin are sensory nerves that can process every sensation from pressure to an annoying itch to serious pain. CBD can have remarkable impacts on this entire ecosystem because skin produces endocannabinoid molecules such as anandamide and 2-AG. These are constantly released, and appear throughout the skin in many different cell types. Endocannabinoids act on receptors such as CB1 and CB2, which are present in all types of skin cells. Thus, CBD can positively change all parts of the skin and help contribute to skin's healthy physiological functions.

Dermatologists have been a little "late to the party" when it comes to CBD research, but the important thing is they're starting to arrive. And the research they *are* doing illustrates that the effects we see on the skin's cannabinoid tone are real.

In "Cannabidiol exerts sebostatic and anti-inflammatory effects on human sebocytes"—published in 2014 in the *Journal of Clinical Investigation*—researchers studied the role of CBD in controlling the inflammation and oiliness of skin. In particular, they were interested in studying the possibility that CBD could be used to treat acne. The researchers administered "CBD to cultured human sebocytes and human skin organ culture inhibited the lipogenic actions of various compounds,

including arachidonic acid and a combination of linoleic acid and testosterone, and suppressed sebocyte proliferation via the activation of transient receptor potential vanilloid-4 (TRPV4) ion channels."

And what were the results of these applications? The researchers found that "CBD behaves as a highly effective sebostatic agent," meaning that it is very effective for treating oily skin. They concluded that "Collectively, our findings suggest that, due to the combined lipostatic, antiproliferative, and anti-inflammatory effects, CBD has potential as a promising therapeutic agent for the treatment of acne vulgaris."

This was pretty strong evidence that CBD could effectively treat acne and/or simple oiliness and inflammation, but the research into CBD and skin was just getting started. Scientists' next target was treating itchy skin.

Activating cannabinoid receptors on certain sensory nerve endings appears to hold the potential to eliminate "false positives" when it comes to skin issues. It's a good thing for our overall health that our skin tells us when we're injured, or when we've come into contact with a contagion or contaminant. However, excessive and unnecessary skin sensation is not something anybody wants and can be a real problem for sufferers. Unpleasant itching is the *most common* reason why Americans see a dermatologist. When there is no underlying reason to the skin's irritation for a physician to correct, CBD may be an excellent choice. The skin's cannabinoid tone can inhibit the spread of pain and thereby ease the body's suffering. In the days ahead, I am confident that we will see CBD deployed more and more as an "anti-itch solution" and as a safe first line of defense for dermatologists to try.

In the 2017 article "The role of cannabinoids in dermatology" published by the *Journal of the American Academy of Dermatology*, the authors explored the promise that CBD holds for "pruritus [itching], inflammatory skin disease, and skin cancer." The authors found that CBD creams have shown qualities to correct many skin conditions, whether they arise from an allergic reaction, injury, or for no specified reason. Their findings determined that "Perhaps the most promising role of cannabinoids is in the treatment of itch." One study on the ability of CBD to correct itch had human test subjects apply cannabinoid cream to itchy areas. Over 86 percent of the study participants said that the cream reduced their itch, and 38 percent said it completely eliminated their itching!

In October 2019, researchers from Johns Hopkins University published an inquiry titled *Cannabinoids for the treatment of refractory chronic pruritus*. This focused specifically on the ability of CBD to positively impact itch alone. Using five different observational studies on the effects of CBD cream on itching, they saw strong evidence of CBD cream effectively treating itching to varying degrees. The authors concluded: "Cannabinoids have the potential to be an effective option in the treatment of chronic pruritus associated with both dermatologic and systemic conditions. The observations made in recent studies require further investigation."

Based upon everything listed above, I think there will be a greater openness on the part of dermatologists to recommend CBD-based skin care products in the future. A recent survey of dermatologists titled "Knowledge, perceptions, and attitudes of cannabinoids in the dermatology community"—published in October 2019 in the *Journal of the American Academy of Dermatology* by researchers from George Washington University—gives me further confidence. They found that 55 percent of dermatologists surveyed said that they had had at least one talk with patients about cannabinoids in the last year. Furthermore, 86 percent said they thought cannabinoids should be legal for medical treatment, and 94 percent said more research should be done on the ability of cannabinoids to help fix skin conditions. Eighty-six percent said they would be willing to prescribe cannabinoids in topical form, and 71 percent said they would prescribe oral cannabinoids. Perhaps most interestingly, 48 percent said that they still worried there could be stigma involved in prescribing cannabinoids to patients. However, that stigma was mostly concentrated in the surveyed dermatologists who were over thirty-five years of age. So as the current generation of dermatologists begins to "move offstage" and a new generation comes to the fore, I expect that dermatologists prescribing CBD-based skin treatments (or recommending over-the-counter versions) will become increasingly common.

In conclusion: using CBD as a topical skin cream is one of the safest and most accessible ways to make CBD part of your daily regimen. In addition to overall skin health and beauty, there is good hard science showing that CBD can be used as an excellent treatment for itching, and to eliminate excessive oil. My one word of caution is this: make sure you know if you have any allergies to the compounds and ingredients that may be used *as part of* the CBD cream. For example, coconut is probably the most popular scent/flavor added to CBD topical cream. (Most CBD creams are scented/flavored.) If your skin has a bad reaction to using the cream, make sure it's not the coconut (or some other ingredient that has been added to the CBD). Generally, consumers do not have skin reactions to CBD alone.

SLEEP

Yawn!

Oh, excuse me. I was just thinking about how millions of my fellow Americans suffer from problems sleeping that go far beyond occasional restlessness. These problems potentially impact many areas of their lives, and in a serious way. From fatigue at work, to inattention, to sexual problems and more, people who have serious trouble sleeping can find their whole lives impacted.

And that's not just my opinion.

According to the CDC, between 30 and 40 percent of Americans regularly struggle to get adequate sleep. Of those Americans who fall into this category, many begin to suffer serious health risk factors. They are more likely to be obese, to be physically inactive, and to smoke or drink excessively. The risks of heart disease, stroke, and even cancer increase along with lack of sleep.

Sleep is also an area where the pharmaceutical industry offers both prescription and over-the-counter aids. Yet many of these are habit-forming, and some can have alarming side effects. For example, according to a July 2018 *Consumer Reports* survey, about 60 percent of people taking traditional sleep medications say that they experience side effects—which can range from sleepiness the next day and feeling confusing or forgetful to so-called "Ambien sleepwalking." In fact, a shocking 3 percent of people using traditional sleep medication report that it has made them fall asleep while driving a vehicle! The same survey also found that many people are likely to find themselves abusing or misusing prescription sleep aids. A concerning 40 percent of respondents said they combine sleep aids with alcohol, or take more than the recommended amount. Many Americans also take prescription sleep aids when they know they will not have time to get 7 or 8 hours of sleep. Because of this, those people are driving or operating machinery with these drugs still impacting and impairing them. A study in the *American Journal of Public Health* found that—as a population—people who take sleep medications are almost twice as likely to be involved in a car accident as people who do not. The same study concluded that people taking sleep aids are as likely to be in a car accident as people who drive while intoxicated.

Enter CBD.

The first thing to say about CBD and sleeplessness is that its ability to treat sleeplessness is probably connected to its ability to treat anxiety, which we've just reviewed. People who are less anxious are able to fall asleep more easily. Therefore, sleeplessness and anxiety are connected.

It is also important to note that better sleep is one of the most prominent things that CBD is known for! In addition to its other benefits, almost everyone taking CBD experiences a better night's sleep. (And there are virtually *zero* reported cases of CBD interrupting or impairing sleep.) Better sleep is also one of the benefits that new users of CBD can experience right away; the effect is often instantaneous. The very day someone uses CBD for the first time, they may report improved sleep that same night. And vitally—unlike most over-the-counter or prescription sleep aids—CBD's effect is usually not to make the user immediately drowsy. Rather, the effect is only felt at the end of the day when the user heads to bed. The reason for this is that CBD is not telling the brain or body that it is time to sleep. Rather, CBD acts by suppressing inflammation, anxiety, and other factors that can keep someone from falling asleep when they are otherwise ready to.

There has been only one prominent hard-science research study using human subjects into the effect of CBD on sleep, but it strongly supports its efficacy. This study, titled "Cannabidiol in Anxiety and Sleep: A Large Case Series," was published in *The Permanente Journal* in 2019. The scientists behind the study took 72 patients as their test subjects, all of whom had anxiety and anxiety-related sleeping issues. The participants were given CBD in capsule form. At the end of the study, the results were clear. Nearly 80 percent of patients reported decreased anxiety, and precisely two-thirds reported improved sleep. The researchers concluded that CBD "may hold benefit" in these areas and urged that additional studies be undertaken.

I strongly suspect that there will be more important studies on CBD and sleep in the years to come. I also project that their results will be similar.

For the moment, to find other "hard science" proof, we have to look to studies on cannabis and sleep. Although these studies involved sleep subjects who had been exposed to both CBD and THC, some researchers in recent years have been attempting to "filter out" what may have been the CBD results in these sleep studies, and which effects came instead from the CBD. For example, a 2017 study published in the medical journal *Current Psychiatry Reports*, titled "Cannabis, Cannabinoids, and Sleep: a Review of the Literature," conducted a comprehensive review of research on cannabis and sleep and attempted to "tease out" the nuances of CBD and THC from the data. They reported that:

> Preliminary research into cannabis and insomnia suggests that cannabidiol (CBD) may have therapeutic potential for the treatment of insomnia. Delta-9 tetrahydrocannabinol (THC) may decrease sleep latency but could impair sleep quality long-term. Novel studies investigating cannabinoids and obstructive sleep apnea suggest that synthetic cannabinoids such as nabilone and dronabinol may have short-term benefit for sleep apnea due to their modulatory effects on serotonin-mediated apneas. CBD may hold promise for REM sleep behavior disorder and excessive daytime sleepiness, while nabilone may reduce nightmares associated with PTSD and may improve sleep among patients with chronic pain. Research on cannabis and sleep is in its infancy and has yielded mixed results. Additional controlled and longitudinal research is critical to advance our understanding of research and clinical implications.

Put plainly, these researchers are saying that the positive effects seen in cannabis and sleep come from the CBD. The THC in cannabis may actually make it more difficult to get a good night's rest. Once again, the experts are identifying CBD as the key.

Some recent medical studies have also mentioned improved sleep as a secondary effect. For example, several medical studies of CBD's ability to control pain have noted—usually as an aside, buried deep in the text—that patients also reported better sleep. Once again,

I believe we are seeing this because CBD positively impacts health issues that tend to be connected. In addition to anxiety, pain is also something that can keep you awake at night when you'd rather be asleep. Eliminate the pain, and you may be well on your way to getting a good night's rest.

And of course, all sleep is not created equal. CBD—you guessed it!—helps there, too.

In 2014, researchers in the Department of Neuroscience and Behavior at the University of São Paulo conducted a study on the impact of CBD on Parkinson's patients. They were performing this test because Parkinson's patients often suffer from disorders impacting REM sleep. In addition to not waking rested, sufferers report increased nightmares and sleepwalking (or similar behaviors). The researchers found that when these patients were given CBD, they had a substantial reduction in sleep-related issues. So here is "proof" that CBD can impact not just quantity, but quality. The Parkinson's patients had been sleeping before their treatment, but sleeping poorly. Now they slept well and without issue.

Despite all this, some researchers have been hesitant to identify CBD as a sleep aid. This is due, partially, to the fact that not enough clinical research exists to back up this statement. Instead, they have said that it shows the potential to eliminate the barriers to a restful night of sleep, and to improve sleep quality. With all due respect, I think that this is debating semantics in a way that most sleepy Americans will not find useful!

Whether CBD truly makes people fall asleep, or just eliminates the barriers to them falling asleep themselves (reduction of inflammation and cortisol), the end result is the same in my book. (And this *is* my book.) CBD has been shown to be non-habit-forming, as some sleep aids clearly have. There are no reported side effects related to feeling groggy the next day, and there are certainly no studies to suggest it increases anybody's chances of being in a car accident or other dangerous situations due to impairment.

CBD impacts everyone differently due to the uniqueness of the endocannabinoid system, and this is also true when it comes to sleep. Good sleep is one of the most common reasons why people use CBD; but each person finds their own route to their best CBD sleep. For example, some people prefer a small dose of CBD to help them fall asleep when they're restless. They feel the effect of the CBD immediately and don't need to take any on nights they don't feel restless. In contrast, other people who use CBD to sleep find that they need to take it every day for several weeks in order to feel the antianxiety and antirestlessness effects that help them sleep. Folks in this category need to take CBD regularly, or else the positive effects on sleep will gradually fade away. CBD is a powerful tool for helping with sleep—but you will have to figure out the optimal use of it, for you personally.

In conclusion, CBD remains the best new hope for treating insomnia affordably, effectively, and with no serious side effects or potential for abuse. And because CBD has the ability to reduce anxiety and stress, which are the most common factors for insomnia, users sleep better almost immediately. I think it is one of the greater benefits that keep CBD users coming back for more.

TOBACCO CESSATION

Another area in which CBD also shows early but considerable promise is in tobacco smoking cessation. Even after decades of informational campaigns alerting consumers to the dangers of cigarettes, smoking still kills about 480,000 Americans each year (about 13 percent of Americans still smoke tobacco). It is the leading cause of preventable death, with nearly one in every five deaths in the USA caused by tobacco use. While great gains have been made in discouraging tobacco use—and helping smokers to quit—these shocking statistics are strong evidence that we still need to do something more.

Maybe that "something more" is CBD.

Since the early 2000s, individual users of CBD have noticed that CBD seems to decrease their urges and gives smokers who've been trying to quit for a while a newfound strength. Research is now beginning to back this observation with hard science.

A 2013 study by the Clinical Psychopharmacology Unit at University College London conducted a double-blind placebo test in which smokers who were trying to quit were given inhalers and encouraged to use them when they

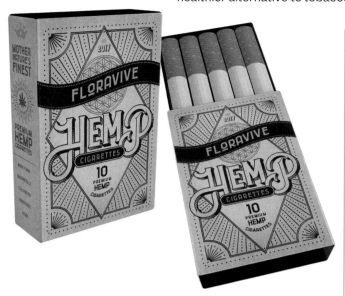

Hemp cigarettes by Floravive gets ahead of the trend with zero chemicals and no synthetics, creating a healthier alternative to tobacco.

shown images known to be smoking cues—such as a photo of a happy person smoking a cigarette—and also control images unrelated to smoking. After each image was shown, the participant was asked to rate how "pleasant" they found it, and to rate it on a scale. When compared to a control group, the researchers found that study participants who had taken a single 800mg dose of CBD before viewing the images were no longer attracted to the smoking-related images, with some even finding them off-putting. Or, as the researchers

felt the urge to smoke. Some of the inhalers contained CBD, while others contained a placebo. Study participants given the placebo showed no reduction in the number of cigarettes smoked. Participants given an inhaler containing CBD smoked an average of 40 percent fewer cigarettes during the course of the study. The researchers concluded that CBD may be a potential treatment for nicotine use and called for additional studies to be conducted.

Another important study on the impact of CBD on smokers was conducted in 2018 by researchers at the same institution and was published in the academic journal *Addiction*. This study involved giving people who were already addicted to cigarettes a dose of CBD at various points and then tested on their "attentional bias" regarding tobacco use cues. For example, a participant in the study would be

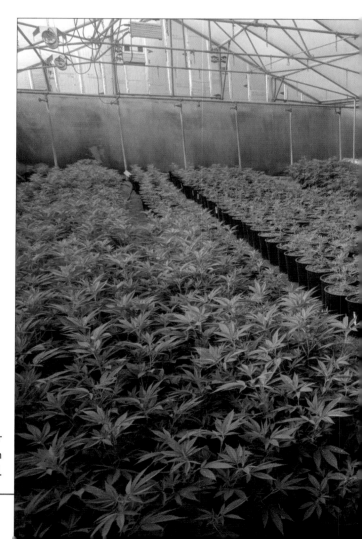

GreenHouse or Indoor Hemp grows are vital to year round farmers in order to keep up with supply and demand.

phrased it, the CBD "reduced explicit pleasantness of cigarette images."

A product that makes you want to smoke 40 percent less and takes away the appeal of the kind of imagery so often found in cigarette advertising? This certainly sounds like it could be a powerful weapon in the arsenal of someone who is trying to improve their health and stop smoking. Though CBD does not appear to be an instant cure for smoking, when used in combination with proven tactics like support groups and replacing "cigarette time" with healthier activities (like taking a walk or participating in a hobby), it seems as though it might definitely be the difference for some smokers.

Now, how exactly does CBD curb the urge to smoke? These are mechanisms that still need to be studied. However, I believe that it is connected to CBD's observed ability to relieve tension, anxiety, and inflammation. How many times do we see a smoker in a stressful situation saying something like: "Gosh, I could use a cigarette"? But using tobacco to address anxiety may be unnecessary if that anxiety has already been addressed by CBD. In addition to anxiety and stress, it is interesting to wonder if there are other physiological elements that can be involved in our ability—or inability—to resist temptation and bad habits. As we learn more about CBD, I continue to wonder if there may be new things we discover about the psychology of addictive behavior and the ability of CBD to act upon it.

If CBD can add years to the lives of countless people around the world by helping them quit smoking, we would be fools not to advocate strongly for its adoption as a go-to solution. For this reason alone, I hope that the millions of smokers across our country will consider giving CBD a chance to help them smoke less or quit entirely.

ALCOHOL ADDICTION

In addition to cigarette smoking, excessive alcohol use is also a serious health problem

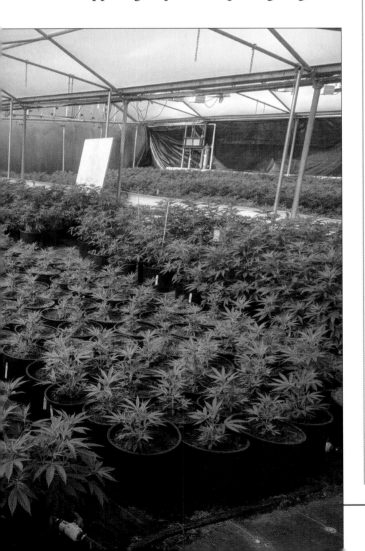

that takes years off the lives of millions of Americans. According to the National Institute of Alcohol Abuse and Alcoholism—which is part of the National Institutes of Health—over half of Americans aged eighteen and older have an alcoholic drink at least once a month. However, about 26 percent of Americans over eighteen engage in potentially dangerous drinking at "binge drinking" levels on a monthly basis. ("Binge drinking" is usually defined as four or more drinks for a woman and five or more drinks for a man.) A certain subset of binge drinkers will go on to develop the most dire form of alcohol use, which the NIH calls "Alcohol Use Disorder." This is defined as "A chronic relapsing brain disease characterized by an impaired ability to stop or control alcohol use despite adverse social, occupational, or health consequences." It is estimated that over 6 percent of all American adults over eighteen have this disorder.

And the effects are plain to see. Nearly 90,000 Americans die from alcohol abuse in the United States each year, making it the third-leading cause of preventable death. It's estimated that the total cost to society of alcohol abuse and misuse might be somewhere around a quarter of a trillion dollars annually. About 30 percent of all fatal car crashes involve an alcohol-impaired driver. One in four college students say that they have had their academic career negatively impacted—which can mean anything from getting a lower grade in a class all the way to failing out of school—because of problematic alcohol misuse. Alcohol misuse by

teenagers in the US kills more teens than does all illegal drug use combined.

Clearly, alcoholism is a serious problem for our country And though there are some systems already in place to treat it, everyone's body is different, and we could benefit from a wider range of solutions. CBD appears to possess several properties that suggest it may be a natural and effective tool for helping even severe alcoholics to transition through withdrawal and make responsible choices.

A 2015 study published in the journal *Substance Abuse* titled "Cannabidiol as an Intervention for Addictive Behaviors: A Systematic Review of the Evidence" sought to evaluate the potential of CBD to fight addiction in humans. The researchers found that CBD had a "beneficial impact" on dependence and concluded it can "be useful in the treatment of addiction disorders" including alcoholism because it "acts on several neurotransmission systems involved in addiction." The authors called for additional research into the addiction-fighting properties of CBD to be conducted.

A 2018 study in *Neuropsychopharmachology* titled "Unique treatment potential of cannabidiol for the prevention of relapse to drug use: preclinical proof of principle" used animal tests to further garner definitive proof of the ability of CBD to help prevent relapse in those who are addicted. The study examined the effect of CBD on both alcohol and cocaine addicts. As the authors themselves put it:

Rats with alcohol or cocaine self-administration

histories received transdermal CBD at 24 h[r] intervals for 7 days and were tested for context and stress-induced reinstatement, as well as experimental anxiety on the elevated plus maze. Effects on impulsive behavior were established using a delay-discounting task following recovery from a 7-day dependence-inducing alcohol intoxication regimen. CBD attenuated context-induced and stress-induced drug seeking without tolerance, sedative effects, or interference with normal motivated behavior. Following treatment termination, reinstatement remained attenuated up to ~5 months although plasma and brain CBD levels remained detectable only for 3 days. CBD also reduced experimental anxiety and prevented the development of high impulsivity in rats with an alcohol dependence history. The results provide proof of principle supporting potential of CBD in relapse prevention along two dimensions: beneficial actions across several vulnerability states and long-lasting effects with only brief treatment.

This study showed that CBD has the power to help reduce alcohol seeking in rats who had been made addicted to alcohol. (While I'm thankful that these studies allow us to make so many important medical strides, let me say here, definitively, that it's frustrating that so much animal testing is conducted. I earnestly hope that in the future—when safe, well-tolerated substances like CBD are tested—animals will not need to be used.)

CBD was effective at deterring the alcoholic rats even when they were placed under stress. Stress is one of the factors that can trigger relapse in alcoholics. Also of note in this study was that CBD, in the words of the researchers, "attenuates drug seeking with effects that far outlast treatment." Put another way, CBD continued to reduce cocaine- and alcohol-seeking behavior in the rats, and this effect continued for some time *even after the rats had stopped taking the CBD*. Though seemingly a small detail, this finding has the potential to inform how CBD can be used to reach people with alcohol addiction disorders. Often, alcoholics (and drug addicts) may not be the most conscientious and responsible people when it comes to remembering to take a pill—such as a pill that reduces cravings. The important finding of this study is that the antirelapse effects of CBD extend beyond the period during which the CBD is taken. So if there is an alcoholic trying not to relapse, and he/she takes CBD in this connection *but* is forgetful and occasionally misses pills, there is good reason to think that the antirelapse effects of the CBD will still be preserved. (Contrast this with a treatment that only works in the twelve or twenty-four hours after a pill is taken. An alcoholic in recovery who forgets or misplaces a single pill could be sent careening back to their addiction immediately.) This study also found that CBD was "devoid of sedative and nonspecific amotivational effects" in the test subjects, meaning that recovering alcoholics taking it would not expect to feel side effects like lethargy.

The conclusions of the authors at the end of the study are especially heartening:

In summary, the results provide proof of principle supporting potential of CBD for relapse prevention along two dimensions: beneficial actions across several vulnerability states, and long-lasting effects with only brief treatment. To further substantiate this putative large-spectrum treatment potential it will be essential to extend the characterization of CBD's "therapeutic" profile in the future. This includes understanding of the post-treatment persistence of CBD's anti-anxiety effects and its efficacy to reduce anxiety in subjects with a history of more excessive, long-term drug use than modeled here. It will be important also to determine the treatment frequency, duration, and doses at which CBD is most efficacious in exerting both its acute and post-treatment "therapeutic" actions. While these issues and the mechanistic basis of CBD's effects require clarification in the future, the results have significant implications concerning CBD's potential in relapse prevention.

They also noted that:

> . . . addicts enter relapse vulnerability states for multiple reasons. Therefore, effects such as these observed with CBD that concurrently ameliorate several of these are likely to be more effective in preventing relapse than treatments targeting only a single state.

Put plainly, the scientists are pointing out that addicts for things like alcohol and cocaine can relapse for a number of different reasons. (Some relapse because of stress, opportunity, peer pressure, boredom, anxiety, physical pain, excitement, or simply for no apparent reason at all.) What is promising about CBD as a potential treatment is that, in addition to being long-lasting, it appears to fight a broad spectrum of addiction triggers. Personally, I think this is not surprising, since those of us in the CBD industry have long known how CBD is liable to impact a large number of areas positively. By cutting stress, pain, inflammation, and impulsive behavior, CBD is likely to help people who are trying to resist an alcohol addiction to stay on the path that leads to recovery and better health and happiness.

Finally, a Canadian study released earlier this year titled "Cannabidiol as a Novel Candidate Alcohol Use Disorder Pharmacotherapy: A Systematic Review" found that previous tests involving cell cultures, animal test subjects, and human test subjects all concluded that "CBD was found to exert a neuroprotective effect against adverse alcohol consequences on the hippocampus." It also found that "CBD attenuates cue-elicited and stress-elicited alcohol seeking, alcohol self-administration, withdrawal-induced convulsions, and impulsive discounting of delayed rewards."

In layman's terms, the Canadian researchers found that a survey of existing studies forced them to conclude that CBD can protect against the negative mental effects of alcohol, while at the same time reducing the urge to drink and also reducing the negative symptoms associated with withdrawal. This newest study builds on the kind of research we saw in the 2018 rat study. By cutting symptoms associated with withdrawal, alcoholics can be less likely to return to drink. Withdrawal symptoms vary widely. They can be as simple as the feeling that you "could really go for a drink right now." However, heavy users who are addicted can suffer extreme symptoms like tremors (or "DTs"), high blood pressure, disorientation, seizures, hallucinations, and powerful feelings of sickness. Quite evidently, those in this latter category will have to do much more than simply "wait until a craving passes." Often, severe withdrawal from alcohol needs to be managed under the care of a physician or other health professional. However, we want alcoholics and those caring for them to have "every tool in the shed" available to help increase the chances of an abuser leaving alcohol behind for good. I think that helping alcoholics to cure themselves is one of the most important and perhaps under-rated opportunities for CBD use. Virtually all of us know someone touched by alcoholism. A key that we all must keep in mind is that it doesn't just affect those who drink. The National Institute of Alcohol Abuse Statistic states that more than 10 percent of all children in the United States are raised by a parent with serious alcohol misuse problems. That impacts countless lives and hurts a vulnerable population. When alcoholics crash cars, start fights, and impact the healthcare system to a great degree, they do more than simply hurt themselves. They hurt society at large and hurt individuals who have never themselves taken a drink. It is tremendously exciting that CBD stands to be a powerful force for fighting this behavior and hopefully improving the quality of life for millions of Americans.

SEVERE MENTAL ILLNESS AND PSYCHOSIS

Let me say at the outset that psychosis and other serious mental illnesses are conditions that should always involve seeking the care of a qualified physician. These conditions can be dire, and a medical professional can always bring a wealth of professional knowledge to the table. Nobody should try to treat their (or a loved one's) serious mental illness themselves.

With that established, it is also important for me to note that there is also ongoing research suggesting that CBD may contain powerful healing properties for those afflicted with mental conditions. If these findings remain consistent—which I fully expect them to—then one day very soon psychiatrists may begin suggesting CBD as a safe, gentle, and non-habit-forming treatment for patients with certain mental conditions.

It's important to frame any discussion of studying CBD's effects on mental illness today with a bit of history. Studies of cannabinoids and their effects on mental illness did not start with the current "CBD boom," and they did not occur in a vacuum. Quite to the contrary: they have always been highly political. The inescapable fact is that for just about all of the twentieth century, the American government has very much wished for any researcher to conclude that cannabinoids *caused* mental illness, as opposed to finding that cannabis could often help to ameliorate the symptoms experienced by the mentally ill. Researchers who reached conclusions that went against the "party line" on cannabis knew that their research funding, teaching positions, and esteem in the scientific community could all be in danger if they published their results. Cannabis was a "gateway drug" that could lead to terrible things, according to the government. Moreover, the government treated drugs as a kind of binary. On one side was "illegal drugs" that had been shown to hurt people. On the other was "medicine" manufactured by the pharmaceutical industry that had been shown to make people better.

I don' t think it is a wild claim or a "conspiracy theory" to imagine that twentieth-century researchers may have ignored results that showed ways in which cannabinoids could help the mentally ill. In fact, our history is full of examples of how the attitude of the American government has had a "chilling effect" on the ability of researchers to uncover the truth and make unbiased, objective discoveries.

To drive the point home, permit me to give you my favorite example of a time when the government's shifting attitudes on substances suppressed important research. It involves no less a personage that our country's founder, George Washington.

In the 1990s, archeologists were studying property that had once been owned by Washington, near his Mt. Vernon estate. Because of Washington's historical importance, his lands had already been studied for decades by other archeologists hoping to uncover new facts about Colonial America and/or our first president. But in the 1990s, a new generation of researchers discovered something strange. On one particular plot of land near Washington's home, there was evidence that excavations had begun . . . but had then abruptly ceased. There was no record as to why the archeological work had been called off, no explanatory notes of the previous generation of researchers. It remained a mystery until those researchers looked at the *dates* of the initial dig on the site. They had been performed in the '20s and '30s . . . during Prohibition.

Historical documents had long referenced Washington as owning a whiskey distilling facility, but nobody had ever found it. When the researchers in the 1990s started digging again, they realized precisely what had happened. Their counterparts seventy years earlier had indeed discovered the ruins of George Washington's distillery. But to report that George Washington himself had been a producer of alcoholic beverages at a time when the nation's government had decided that alcohol should be banned would have been controversial to say the least! Likely afraid of losing their government funding, the archeologists of yore had simply covered over their discovery and falsified their notes. (New excavations were eventually undertaken, and it was revealed that Washington owned one of the largest distilleries in the United States, producing over 11,000 gallons a year at its peak! In 2007, the distillery was rebuilt and is now a tourist attraction operated by the government.)

Washington's distillery may be an extreme example, but it shows how the prevailing attitudes held by the government—and/or by a majority of its citizens—can impact and skew the results of scientific research.

For much of the twentieth century, with cannabinoids classified as a "bad drug" by those in power—and presented as almost tantamount to substances like cocaine and heroin—researchers studying cannabis almost always published research showing that it *caused* mental illness. Today, we are better able to view these older findings in their proper context. What most twentieth-century researchers *actually* found was that cannabis presented *no serious health dangers or side effects*. What they emphasized to the public was a finding at the extreme edge of the spectrum, namely, that very heavy users of THC could sometimes experience psychosis, psychosis-like symptoms, or other cognitive impairments. In my opinion, emphasizing only the results of very heavy THC use was disingenuous. It would be like researchers claiming to study the effects of alcohol, then omitting all findings that showed moderate consumption was safe (or, in the case of red wine, possible beneficial) and sharing only the health results of severe alcoholics who engaged in constant binge drinking.

Now, however, the pendulum is beginning to swing back in the other direction when it comes to our attitudes about cannabinoids. And thank goodness that it is, because it looks like they have a *tremendous* amount of relief to offer people who struggle with mental illness.

Researchers studying cannabis in the twenty-first century have found that cannabinoids can actually help to reduce the symptoms of mental illness in many cases. And while extremely high amounts of THC in cannabis have been shown to cause mental impairment, cannabis with large amounts of CBD have been shown to correct it.

A 2011 study in the journal *Schizophrenia Research* titled "Cannabis with high cannabidiol content is associated with fewer psychotic experiences" found that while historically, "cannabis is associated with psychotic outcomes in numerous studies . . . there are an increasing number of authors who identify cannabidiol [CBD] as an antipsychotic agent." The authors surveyed records of 1,877 cannabis users who used different strains of cannabis and who, in some cases, had reported on growing or lessening psychotic symptoms. Lo and behold, the researchers found that there was a direct relationship between using cannabis with higher CBD content and a lessening of psychotic symptoms. The researchers concluded that "using high cannabidiol content cannabis was associated with significantly lower degrees of psychotic symptoms." They noted that their findings would be augmented by more studies into how CBD could help the mentally ill. This 2011 study was the largest and most comprehensive when it was conducted, but other scientists and physicians had already been undertaking smaller-scale work on the positive impact of CBD on patients with psychosis. As far back as the 1990s, forward-thinking doctors had been looking at ways CBD could be useful in this area.

In 1995, the article "Antipsychotic effects of cannabidiol" was published in the *Journal of Clinical Psychiatry*. It is thought to be the very first published report on an MD treating a patient with CBD. In the study, a young woman with a diagnosis of schizophrenia was given 1500mg of CBD over a four-week period, which resulted in a considerable improvement of her most extreme symptoms. While the 1995 study was only one physician sharing good results with the rest of the medical community, it helped put CBD on the map a little bit and may have led other doctors to consider such treatment as a viable option for similar patients. In addition, it helped researchers who were starting to look at CBD for *other* conditions stop and notice when it presented additional antipsychotic effects. Suddenly, researchers and physicians all over the place were finding that CBD could control psychotic symptoms as an added benefit to an already impressive array of potential benefits.

In 2012, researchers at the University of São Paulo and the National Institute for Translational Medicine were publishing findings suggesting that CBD was able to comport powerful antipsychotic effects on patients in clinical trials. Though the Brazilian researchers did not, at that time, fully understand the mechanism by which CBD was producing these positive results (currently we would point to its antiinflammatory properties), the researchers suggested that new studies should be undertaken and that CBD could be a powerful tool for treating psychosis, especially schizophrenia.

Also in 2012, another team of researchers conducted the first large-scale, double-blind randomized trial on the effects of CBD on controlling psychotic symptoms. Published in the journal *Translational Psychiatry*, the research—titled "Cannabidiol enhances anandamide signaling and alleviates psychotic symptoms of schizophrenia"—showed that individuals who had been diagnosed with schizophrenia saw a benefit to taking CBD in the form of symptom reduction. In this study, the test subjects were given 600–800mg of CBD for a month. As a means of contrast, another group in the study was given amisulpride. (Often known under the brand name Solian, amisulpride is an FDA-approved antipsychotic medicine commonly used to treat schizophrenia.) The researchers in this study found that the CBD was just as effective as the FDA-approved amisulpride in reducing the symptoms of schizophrenia, *and also* that CBD had far fewer side effects experienced by the subjects (if they experienced any at all). As the researchers concluded:

Our results provide evidence that the non-cannabimimetic constituent of marijuana, cannabidiol, exerts clinically relevant antipsychotic effects that are associated with marked tolerability and safety, when compared with current medications. Although a plethora of pharmacological mechanisms have recently been suggested relevant for the antipsychotic effect of cannabidiol the primary pharmacological mechanism through which cannabidiol exerts this antipsychotic effect in humans is unclear at present. [. . .] Nevertheless, our results do provide a rationale for additional clinical testing of selective FAAH inhibitors in schizophrenia.

A pretty strong endorsement, with all the caveats we have come to expect regarding CBD. While the researchers acknowledge that the precise mechanism by which CBD works is still unknown, the fact is that it works—and it works with virtually no serious side effects. (Amisulpuride, on the other hand, though effective, can often cause muscle tremors and significant weight gain, among other side effects.)

Another important study was published in 2017 in the *American Journal of Psychiatry*. This work, titled "Cannabidiol (CBD) as an Adjunctive Therapy in Schizophrenia: A Multicenter Randomized Controlled Trial," saw CBD studied in a large-scale double-blind test when it was given to people who suffer from schizophrenia *in addition to* their normal medications. This was such an important study because it answered questions about a scenario that might likely occur in real-world treatment. Namely, a physician has heard about the promising effects of CBD but does not want to take his or her patient off their current meds; what

is likely to happen if CBD is simply added *in addition to* their current medication?

Participants in this study were given either 1000mg of CBD daily or a placebo and continued to take their regular antipsychotic medication(s). After six weeks, the results were tabulated and checked. They showed that patients who took the CBD—not the placebo—had "lower levels of positive psychotic symptoms" and "were more likely to have been rated as improved." Most exciting of all, the patients who took the CBD had only mild side effects, and those occurred at a rate and level of severity that was identical to those who took the placebo. In their conclusion, the researchers noted:

These findings suggest that CBD has beneficial effects in patients with schizophrenia. As CBD's effects do not appear to depend on dopamine receptor antagonism, this agent may represent a new class of treatment for the disorder.

This second sentence was extremely important to other researchers who had been looking into CBD. That's because it found that CBD did not interact adversely with the current, dopamine receptor-based antipsychotic medications that the test subjects were already taking. In addition, they concluded that CBD apparently attacked the symptoms of the condition in an entirely new way. This meant that such treatments could probably be "stacked" on top of other treatments, with no loss of effectiveness for either. Essentially, it provided a new set of clues about how CBD might work.

Other studies around the same time have further refined our knowledge of what CBD can or can't do for patients suffering from mental illness.

The 2018 study "The effects of cannabidiol (CBD) on cognition and symptoms in outpatients with chronic schizophrenia a randomized placebo controlled trial" published in *Psychopharmacology* set out to specifically study the impact of CBD on cognition in people with schizophrenia. Study participants were given 600mg of CBD daily—or a placebo—and their cognitive performances were studied. However, at the end of the research, the scientists found that schizophrenic patients who had taken the CBD did not show an improvement in cognition when compared with those who had taken the placebo. Or, as they put it: "At the dose studied, CBD augmentation was not associated with an improvement in MCCB or PANSS scores in stable antipsychotic-treated outpatients with schizophrenia." I think studies like this are important, even when they're used to show what CBD *cannot* do for a certain ailment or population. There's so much evidence for the good things that CBD does that there's certainly no reason to feel threatened or downcast when it is shown not to work on something. (In fact, so many of CBD's results are so very positive for beneficial effects that having studies like this tends to lend more credence to the overall conversation around CBD. When something shows too many successes with too few side effects, we fall back to that "too good to be true" fallacy.

And that's another way the public, the government, and some in the scientific community continue to resist CBD.)

Precisely how and why CBD can have positive effects on people with mental illness is the last frontier of this inquiry. We know that CBD doesn't bind with cannabinoid receptors in the same way THC does, and we know that it can probably interact with anandamide at a cellular level. CBD may be a useful treatment for mental illness because of how it impacts levels of anandamide, but more research is needed in this area. There are currently multiple active trials happening all over the globe to test the impacts of CBD.

In conclusion, CBD's positive impact on mental illness is promising and exciting. Not only that, but it also represents a great case study to help cannabinoids move away from the tainted and skewed "research" that emerged during much of the twentieth century and reframe CBD as the promising and safe cure that it is.

Let me state again that anybody dealing with a serious mental condition should seek the help of a professional.

The research studies thus far are as clear as they can be: CBD is effective at controlling many of the major symptoms of mental illnesses, like psychosis. CBD has virtually no negative side effects for patients who take it for these symptoms, and does not negatively interact with the existing antipsychotic medicines that have been studied. In fact, research suggests that CBD may be able to augment *existing* meds, as it comes at the problem from an entirely different "point of attack."

If you're seeing a physician for help with a mental illness and they have not brought up CBD as a treatment possibility, don't hesitate to lend them this book or cite for them the studies in this section. You may be glad you did.

INJURY

Our bodies are remarkable machines in many ways, but perhaps nothing is more awe-inspiring than the complicated and ingenious ways our bodies can heal themselves. If you've ever cut yourself, broken a bone, or hit your head, wounds and injuries involve more than the simple tear or break we have sustained. Our wounds swell and turn colors, we feel pain, we feel lethargic. Much of this is caused by inflammation, and while some may be useful to the healing process, excessive inflammation is not.

Inflammation during injuries is part of our body's response to molecular patterns associated with the release of dead and dying cells, and also sometimes from infection. Injuries involve complex inflammatory responses that accompany the body in repairing itself. These inflammations aren't a bad thing on their own per se, but they shouldn't be allowed to persist longer than needed.

Our immune systems responds to injuries and inflammation in a number of ways, and our endocannabinoid system is key in regulating immune responses. Most of its work is immunosuppressive, which is where CBD can come in, as its properties are about to help regulate healing to make it more effective, less painful for the patient, and allow it to occur without unnecessary inflammation.

Therapeutic strategies, I believe, can be derived from this knowledge. We know that CBD impacts inflammation, and we have seen that it can have likewise positive impacts on our immune systems. This is definitely an area where further research is still needed. Both the immune system and the endocannabinoid system play crucial roles in helping us recover from injuries, and when these roles can be more fully understood, I believe physicians will realize that they have a new and satisfying option for helping patients recover from injuries more effectively and with less inflammation and pain.

A study published in 2015 in the *Journal of Bone and Mineral Research* found that CBD sped up the healing of bone fractures. The study—conducted by researchers from several institutions around the world—tested both the effects of CBD and THC on healing fractures. Ultimately, the researchers found that while CBD had healing benefits, THC did not. The researchers were excited by their findings, not only for the promise they held in developing tools to heal broken bones, but also for treating bone-related diseases like osteoporosis. As Dr. Yankel Gabet, one of the authors of the study said, in a press announcement:

The clinical potential of cannabinoid-related compounds is simply undeniable at this point. While

THE SCIENCE OF CANNABIS

Aids sleep
Fights free radicals
in the blood stream
Relaxes muscles

Relieves pain
Boosts relaxation
Slows inflammation

Encourages cell growth
Stops fungus growth

TETRAHYDOCANNABINOL

Stimulates
bone growth

CANNABINOL

the

CANNABICHROMENE

Reduces
risk of nerve
damage

cbn

cbc

CANNABIGEROL

cbg

cbd

CANNABIDIOL

thev

Stops bacteria growth
Boosts cell growth

TETRAHYDOCANNABIVARIN

Boosts
appetite

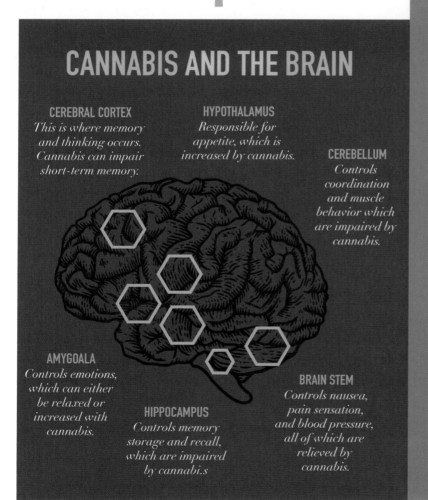

CANNABIS AND THE BRAIN

CEREBRAL CORTEX
This is where memory and thinking occurs. Cannabis can impair short-term memory.

HYPOTHALAMUS
Responsible for appetite, which is increased by cannabis.

CEREBELLUM
Controls coordination and muscle behavior which are impaired by cannabis.

AMYGOALA
Controls emotions, which can either be relaxed or increased with cannabis.

HIPPOCAMPUS
Controls memory storage and recall, which are impaired by cannabi.s

BRAIN STEM
Controls nausea, pain sensation, and blood pressure, all of which are relieved by cannabis.

NEUROLOGICAL

Can inhibit tumor growth

May reduce migraine
frequency & intensity

Helps control epileptic seizures

May slow the progression of Alzheimer's

OPTHALMOLOGICAL

Reduces glaucoma symptoms

PSYCHOLOGICAL

Can promote better sleep

Helps manage bipolar disorder

Eases anxiety

Treats depression

Can help treat depression and PTSD

Helps manage ADD and ADHD

ABDOMINAL

Can relieve chronic symptons of
IBD and Crohn's disease

Helps treat incontinence

Eases symptons of PMS

Stimulates appetite

PALLIATIVE CARE

Eases chemotherapy side effects

Reduces chronic pain

May improve bone health

there is still a lot of work to be done to develop appropriate therapies, it is clear that it is possible to detach a clinical therapy objective from the psychoactivity of cannabis. CBD, the principal agent in our study, is primarily anti-inflammatory and has no psychoactivity. [. . .] We found that CBD alone makes bones stronger during healing, enhancing the maturation of the collagenous matrix, which provides the basis for new mineralization of bone tissue. After being treated with CBD, the healed bone will be harder to break in the future. [. . .] We found CBD alone to be sufficiently effective in enhancing fracture healing. Other studies have also shown CBD to be a safe agent, which leads us to believe we should continue this line of study in clinical trials to assess its usefulness in improving human fracture healing.

Healing bones is among the most ancient tasks for physicians, so perhaps it makes sense that we are now finding that one of our most ancient drugs helps the process! The proof that CBD can help with bone healing has inspired additional research into the underpinnings of CBD's ability to help our body repair itself and recover from injury (and prevent reinjury). And more recent studies have pointed to the remarkable fact that CBD does not seem to interact in a negative way when physicians need to administer other drugs as part of the healing process.

For example, an interesting study conducted by researchers in Texas in 2019 looked at users of CBD who were treated in hospitals for psychiatric conditions—specifically at length of hospital stays. Generally, when treatments go well, a person is quickly discharged from the hospital. A longer hospital stay, on the other hand, can indicate difficulties with treatment, complications, or longer healing times. The Texas study found that patients who regularly used CBD did not take any longer to treat or heal than non-CBD users.

While this was not as groundbreaking as the bone study, I include it here to note that CBD did not hinder healing in any way when it came to mental conditions. A study like this one could be undertaken to examine the effect of CBD on people in hospitals recovering from physical injuries, and I'd be willing to bet that we'd see some very interesting results.

A large amount of hard (and anecdotal) evidence about CBD's ability to help with healing has emerged from the physical fitness community. Athletes are always looking for something to give them an "edge." For professional athletes competing at the highest levels, even small improvements can prove vital in competition. When it comes to the career of an athlete, the ability to recover from injuries, competitions, and difficult workouts can be the difference between making the team or getting cut.

Athletes have historically not been shy about exploring whether supplements and medicines might be able to improve some aspect of their performance. (There is not enough room here to adequately go into the history of athletes who have skirted the law to "up their game," but you only have to look at the headlines to see how prevalent it is—and it starts early in life. According to the Mayo Clinic, an estimated 5 percent of all high school athletes have used anabolic steroids.)

But what if there were a supplement that helped athletes heal and that was not only effective, but completely legal and safe? It's really no wonder that the physical fitness community has been among the first to discover the benefits of using CBD. Though frustratingly, not all of the pro sports leagues have taken an enlightened view on the subject.

While the NFL currently has a medical committee looking into the potential of CBD as a therapy for its athletes, it currently prohibits the substance, as do the NBA, NHL, and MLB. (The PGA and pro tennis, however, do allow CBD use.) Athletes in leagues where CBD is banned can face fines, suspensions, and even dismissal. CBD is viewed as a performance-enhancing drug. This is more than a little frustrating. Many pro sports teams claim to care about the health of their athletes, and yet they ban a substance that holds a real potential to help their players stay healthy and safe. At the same time, the amount of opioids supplied to professional athletes is astounding. Yet losing this customer base would be a huge blow for the pharmaceutical companies. Because of the powerful forces involved in this dynamic, I think that we can expect changes in these policies to come slowly . . . when they come at all.

Athletes who play and train hard often experience soreness, which can be severe. Muscles can swell and tear and become damaged in other ways—all in the course of regular athletic competition. Because of CBD's anti-inflammatory properties, it can have immediate positive impact on athletes. Taking CBD to reduce inflammation can help with muscle recovery and may allow on-the-field injuries to begin healing quicker. In addition, as all athletes learn, sleep is vital for keeping in top shape; muscles do not recover properly after a workout if one does not get adequate sleep or sleeps poorly. Because of this, many athletes have discovered that a safe sleep aid like CBD does wonders for their rest and muscle recovery. There's also a good deal of anecdotal evidence that CBD can help athletes perform better by reducing pain. Most professionals (at all levels) dislike over-the-counter or prescription pain solutions because they can have side effects, such as making them feel logy or run-down. (In addition, many leagues have strict drug policies, and many of these over-the-counter supplements can cause positive drug tests. Furthermore, many professional athletes run the risk of becoming addicted to opioids during their playing careers.) Taking CBD can help to ease the aches and pains involved in training and competition, without the side effects or dangers that can come with other meds. CBD can be taken orally for pain, or a CBD cream can be applied to the site of an inflammation or painful area directly. Athletes have many options when it comes to how to apply the treatment.

Though it is not related to healing and pain per se, I should note here that many athletes also find CBD beneficial because of its helpfulness with anxiety, as we reviewed in a previous section. No matter how much an athlete prepares, almost everyone suffers from "game day jitters." In extreme cases, this competition-related anxiety goes beyond mere excitement and actually effects the player's performance in a negative way. Traditional anxiety medications often have sedative properties, which would be completely counterproductive for an athlete to take before a game. However, use of CBD—either regularly, as part of a training routine, or taken only just before "the big game"—can help players to lose the negative consequences of anxiety without hurting their athletic ability or clear-headedness. I hope that the major pro sports leagues will soon see the wisdom of allowing players to take advantage of these safe and effective solutions.

Many athletes also concentrate on "recovery time" between games or workouts. For a professional athlete, having a short recovery time can be essential for maintaining a successful career. Injuries like muscle tears, sprained and twisted ankles, and dislocations are all common hurdles they must face. These are another example of an area where a player who can recover more quickly can boost his or her value. Every injury is unique, but a player who can generally recover from a sprained ankle in half the time of their counterpart is going to make themselves a hot commodity.

For the most dangerous and punishing sports of all, there is evidence that CBD can even be lifesaving!

A 2014 study by researchers at UCLA titled "Effect of marijuana use on outcomes in traumatic brain injury" examined large populations of people who had suffered traumatic brain injuries, also known as TBIs. It found that people who used cannabis had a 5 to 6 percent greater chance of surviving a TBI than nonusers. The study did not differentiate between the positive effects of THC versus CBD among survivors. However, given what we know so far, there is very little reason to suspect it was the THC—and very considerable reason to suspect it was the CBD—that produced this result in the cannabis users.

Many of the most popular sports today are among the most dangerous and the most likely to involve head injuries. From car racing to boxing to football to ice hockey, thousands upon thousands of athletes take on the risk of a head injury as part of the risk involved in pursuing their athletic passion. Nonetheless, businesses, athletic trainers, and physicians are constantly pursuing innovations that can reduce the risk to competitors. Just consider the evolution in football helmets since the leatherhead days of the 1930s, or the vast number of safety improvements made to race cars. If CBD is even able to add a *small* safety benefit to athletes competing in the most dangerous sports, then it would be irresponsible *not* to examine adopting it across the board.

If you're an athlete at any level, looking into the benefits of CBD can be a wise idea—as long as it is permitted in the league where you play. At the very least, there's good evidence you'll feel less pain after workouts, suffer from less inflammation, and recover from injuries more quickly. At the other extreme, there's a very real chance that CBD can help an elite athlete bolster a pro career or prove to be life-saving in the most dangerous of sports.

I believe that CBD in terms of physical injuries is going to be a very important field of research in the very near future—if only from the money to be made. The global market for sports drinks is nearly $30 billion. The physical therapy industry stands at about $34 billion annually. And the revenue created by professional sports *in North America alone* is about $75 billion per year. As CBD is shown to be a real game-changer in healing, recovery, and injury reduction, I hope that the powerful forces currently skeptical about its use will be forced to "see the light" and come around. At the same time, if additional studies show CBD helps to do things like heal broken bones, orthopedists may start suggesting it for those nonprofessional athletes among us, as well.

MIGRAINE HEADACHES

While we have all had headaches in our life, migraines are a very specific type that can be very serious and very painful. Ask anyone who has had one, and they'll tell you that they're willing to try just about anything to make them stop.

Migraine headaches (or just migraines) are often accompanied by extreme sensitivity to light and sound. For reasons still not fully understood, severe migraines can sometimes cause sufferers to see "cracks" or "jagged lines" of light. If untreated, they can be absolutely debilitating for the sufferer—who may not be able to work, socialize, or engage in other typical activities during the duration of a headache. The cause of migraines is not known, nor is their purpose (if one exists). Traumatic brain injuries can sometimes lead to migraines, but they are more commonly genetic in origin (and often inherited from generation to generation).

Current theories run that the onset of a migraine can be triggered by an interaction between the trigeminal nerve and the brain stem. Others think that serotonin may be involved.

For many years, there were no effective treatments for migraines. Sufferers were generally told to do the kinds of things that can help with general health—get enough sleep, exercise, eat a healthy diet, avoid drinking to excess and smoking, and so forth.

In the middle of the twentieth century, physicians and scientists began developing migraine treatments that proved more effective. In the late twentieth and early twenty-first centuries, this resulted in prescription medications that have given at least some sufferers relief. However, most of the prescription medicines for migraine headaches also have the potential for serious side effects. In addition, patients are often tempted to take too much of these drugs, which can result in a condition called "rebound headaches," which cause the headache to "rebound" when the ever-increasing dose wears off.

The journey of a typical migraine sufferer today involves starting with over-the-counter medications, possibly looking for homeopathic solutions online, and eventually going to a physician for a powerful prescription medicine (and bracing themselves for the possibility of powerful side effects).

But it may not have to be this way.

Groundbreaking studies have already shown that there is likely a link between migraines and the endocannabinoid system and that CBD may have the real potential to bring relief to migraine sufferers in a safer and more effective way than has yet been tried.

The first study to which I'm referring appeared just over a decade ago in the journal *Therapeutics and Clinical Risk Management*. It was titled "Cannabinoids in the management of difficult to treat pain" and was written by Dr. Ethan Russo. In this work, Dr. Russo studied the effects of cannabinoids to treat pain via the endocannabinoid system, with an eye to exploring the growing crisis of unaddressed chronic pain. Dr. Russo posited that some difficult-to-manage pain—such as migraines—may arise from an endocannabinoid deficiency that treatment with cannabinoids would be likely to address. This deficiency would explain why pain, for some patients, has been notoriously difficult to treat. Russo not only found that cannabinoids were likely to be an excellent choice for this kind of pain, but also that the adjacent effects of use could be beneficial for many people. As Russo concluded:

Cannabinoids may offer significant "side benefits" including analgesia. These include anti-emetic effects, well established with THC, but additionally demonstrated for CBD (Pertwee 2005), the ability of THC and CBD to produce apoptosis in malignant cells and inhibit cancer-induced angiogenesis (Kogan 2005; Ligresti et al. 2006), as well as the neuroprotective antioxidant properties of the two substances (Hampson et al. 1998), and improvements in symptomatic insomnia (Russo et al. 2007).

The degree to which cannabinoid analgesics will be adopted into adjunctive pain management practices currently remains to be determined . . . [However,] given their multi-modality effects upon various nociceptive pathways, their adjunctive side benefits, the efficacy and safety profiles to date of specific preparations in advanced clinical trials, and the complementary mechanisms and advantages of their combination with opioid therapy, the future for cannabinoid therapeutics appears very bright, indeed.

Research building upon this work by Dr. Russo was then published in 2014 by a team of researchers in the *Journal of Headache Pain*. The article, "Activation of CB2 receptors as a potential therapeutic target for migraine: evaluation in an animal model," reported on their work using lab rats to test the ability of cannabinoids to address a migraine headache such as might arise from an endocannabinoid deficiency by acting on CB2 receptors. While I find experiments on animals distasteful, these results were truly helpful to understanding how the endocannabinoid system works:

In the present study, we have shown that activation of CB2 receptor, by means of AM1241 administration, induces analgesia [pain killing] . . . The present study lends further support to the therapeutic potential in migraine of probes that interfere with the endocannabinoid system. More specifically, stimulation of CB2 receptors seems promising as it counteracts NTG-induced hyperalgesia in phase II of the formalin test and it is theoretically less likely to induce CNS side effects. However, the impact of long-term treatment with CB2 agonists on their anti-hyperalgesic efficacy and on their effect on the immune system function remains to be elucidated.

This is truly exciting stuff. There may be an entire category of migraine headaches caused by a deficiency that was never properly understood until now and that we may be able to remedy with the application of a safe and plentiful natural substance.

But we're not done yet.

A 2017 study published by the *European Academy of Neurology* titled "Cannabinoids suitable for migraine prevention" offers even more definitive proof that we are on the right track. The first part of this study was conducted on human subjects who suffered from migraines and cluster headaches (a somewhat similar condition, and often even more painful). Subjects were given varying combinations of THC and CBD. It was found that when the concentrations of CBD and THC were high enough, acute pain suffered by the test subjects declined by an average of 55 percent. In the second phase of the study, patients were given either a CBD–THC combination or the leading prescription medication for their condition (migraines or cluster headaches). And again, the results were very encouraging. After a three-month treatment period, the migraine patients on CBD–THC saw a 40.4 percent reduction in migraines, while those on the leading prescription medication saw a reduction of 40.1 percent. Clearly, the cannabinoids were as effective as prescription medication. Unfortunately, the researchers reported that "the severity and number of cluster headache attacks only fell slightly" with the CBD–THC, unless those cluster headache sufferers "had experienced migraine in childhood." At the end of the paper, the researchers concluded definitively: "We were able to demonstrate that cannabinoids are an alternative to established treatments in migraine prevention." However, unfortunately for sufferers, they may not be useful for cluster headaches:

1. Of all the serious medical conditions profiled in this section, there may be none more promising for effective future treatment by CBD than migraine headaches. In a field where there are so many experiments yet to be performed, this is a rare case where we can pretty much say: we know why cannabinoids work for this ailment;

2. We know that they work on animals; and

3. We know that they work for humans.

If you suffer from migraine headaches, the treatment possibilities offered by CBD could not be clearer or more immediately accessible. If you work with a physician, you can also talk with them about trying CBD for your migraine headaches along with any prescription medications you may have been given.

ASTHMA

The interaction between cannabis and asthma has been studied for many decades, and there is very recent research strongly suggesting that cannabinoids might be able to help people in need of improved bronchodilation. (Bronchodilation simply means the expansion of air passages through the bronchi of the lungs during the act of breathing.) These findings will have the potential to help people with asthma and other forms of lung disease.

Unfortunately, asthma research is a topic that was clouded for generations by the "War on Drugs." Because cannabis was on the government's hit list, most of the research went into studying how it might *aggravate* your asthma if you smoked it, as opposed to medicinal uses. The government rewarded research that showed how consuming cannabis by smoking marijuana could *trigger* an asthma attack, which became just another piece of information they could point to under the header "Why you shouldn't do drugs."

But a few enterprising researchers—while acknowledging that smoking cannabis (or smoking anything) could certainly be a bad idea for people with asthma—began also pointing out that there were other ways in which patients could consume cannabinoids. Ways that *didn't* involve smoking.

Might it be possible, they asked, for cannabinoids consumed without smoke to have a different sort of impact on cannabis users . . . perhaps even a positive one?

Despite the war on drugs being in full force during the Regan administration, in 1984 the journal *Clinical Pharmacology & Therapeutics* published a very important study titled "Acute and subacute bronchial effects of oral cannabinoids." In this study, subjects were given a wide variety of cannabinoids—including CBD and THC—in oral form (not inhaled). The effects of bronchodilation on test subjects was observed. The researchers concluded that some cannabinoids did indeed seem to produce "bronchodilator activity." This activity, they deduced, might have the potential to help treat asthma.

Despite being an early study—and one that presented very tentative findings—the first shot had been fired, so to speak. The scientific community had affirmed that they were not only going to investigate how cannabis smoke could aggravate asthma, they were also going to look at how cannabinoids taken in other ways might help asthmatics.

The next major study on cannabinoids and asthma emerged over a decade later, in the journal *Nature*. In 2000, a team of researchers from Hungary, Italy, and the United States published "Bidirectional control of airway responsiveness by endogenous cannabinoids," which was an examination of the ability of cannabinoids to inhibit bronchospasms. Though not focused on CBD, the study found that anandamide could control spasms, which could lead to coughing or even asthma attacks. In the study, subjects had their throats intentionally irritated by a mild chemical so as to induce a cough response. When treated with anandamide, the urge to cough was significantly repressed. The researchers thought this might be additional evidence that cannabinoids could be useful in treating a number of conditions, including asthma and the coughing fits that can trigger such an attack. As the researchers put it: "Our results may account for the contrasting bronchial actions of cannabis-like drugs in humans, and provide a framework for the development of more selective cannabinoid-based agents for the treatment of respiratory pathologies."

In 2015, *Bioorganic & Medicinal Chemistry* published "Cannabidiol (CBD) and its analogs: a review of their effects on inflammation." This paper provided additional information for those interested in CBD for asthma treatment, as it found data that strongly hinted that CBD could be useful in treating many of the symptoms and causes of lung disease due to the fact that it reduced the production of cytokines and chemokines, which cause inflammation in the lungs.

Another important research piece from 2015 was "Evaluation of Serum Cytokines Levels and the Role of Cannabidiol Treatment

in Animal Model of Asthma," published by a group of Brazilian scientists in the journal *Mediators of Inflammation*. Though an animal study, the work had exciting implications for humans. Seeking to explore the interactions of T cells with inflammation, the researchers investigated the ability of CBD to control inflammatory asthma responses in rats. The rats were given regular doses of CBD and then administered "aerosol challenges" to simulate the effects of asthma. The results were remarkable! The rats that had been treated with CBD had much better controlled asthma responses. As the researchers declared:

> We here demonstrate a protective effect of CBD upon inflammatory response in an animal model of asthma; both Th1 and Th2 responses are blunted by CBD treatment. [. . .] The protective effects of CBD upon lung inflammation were demonstrated in several different models. [. . .] In humans, several attempts to decrease inflammatory response in asthma have been tested. Anti-interleukin-4 and anti-interleukin-5 had been effective in reducing exacerbations and persistent eosinophilia in asthmatic patients. In addition, anti-interleukin-9 and anti-interleukin-13 decreased symptoms associated with asthma. In this context, since CBD was used safely in humans, it is possible to suggest that a rapid transition to study its effects in humans is possible.

In plain English, the Brazilian researchers were saying, "We've definitely proven that CBD helps prevent asthma attacks in rats, and so there's no reason we shouldn't rapidly move to prove that it also works in humans."

Then in 2019, a team of researchers published the definitive human study "Cannabidiol reduces airway inflammation and fibrosis in experimental allergic asthma" in the *European Journal of Pharmacology*. This study used human subjects to test the effectiveness of CBD on treating the chronic lung inflammation and airway hyper-responsiveness that characterize asthma. The results were striking, with the researchers finding that "CBD treatment, regardless of dosage, decreased airway hyper-responsiveness." The scientists had noticed that even a small amount of CBD was able to effectively treat the irritation and can over-trigger the normal airway response and cause asthmatic symptoms and an asthmatic attack.

As so often seems to be the case with the most exciting areas of CBD study, much research into CBD remains ongoing; physicians and scientists around the world are continuing to do additional tests and studies. So the question should be asked: where do things stand for someone who currently has asthma and is interested in a CBD-based treatment? Well, down the road I think if research continues to show the dramatically positive ability of CBD to act on inflammation (and for cannabinoids to serve as a bronchodilator), it's likely that the pharmaceutical industry will develop a CBD (or some other cannabinoid formulation) Inhaler for people with asthma. Until that happens, people seeking to ward off the effects of lung and bronchial inflammation

may do well to take regular doses of CBD in order to reduce general inflammation.

UPSET STOMACH AND NAUSEA

Most of the time, feeling sick to your stomach is a symptom, not a disease or condition. It's just your body telling you that something is wrong. You could be injured, sick, or have consumed something poisonous. These causes of nausea can usually be addressed. However, millions of Americans must deal with nausea that cannot be corrected because it is caused by side effects from prescription medication. Nausea can be mild, serious, or anywhere in between. "Curing" nausea has long been a goal of physicians, back to the earliest days of medicine. Over the centuries, effective and safe medications began to be developed to help people deal with especially severe nausea. Some anti-nausea medications are particular to a type of nausea—such as motion sickness. Others are more general in the types of illnesses to which they may be applied. In most cases, patients taking medicine to fight nausea must try different medications and find the one that fits them best.

For many years, anecdotal evidence has existed that states that cannabis could be used to effectively treat nausea. People who were undergoing chemotherapy and people who were suffering from the effects of HIV/AIDS found that using cannabis greatly reduced their stomach sickness and urge to vomit. In fact, the use of cannabis for these patients became one of the most persuasive arguments for legalizing medical marijuana in many states. The hard science that backed up the claims from cannabis users also helped lead to the development of cannabis-based prescription drugs such as Dronabinol, which is approved by the FDA for the treatment of nausea in people undergoing cancer treatment or living with HIV/AIDS. Dronabinol has been available in the marketplace since the 1990s, and it was a powerful test case for proving that FDA-approved drugs made with cannabinoids could be used safely and would not create a spike in drug addiction or misuse. An article published in the *Journal of Psychoactive Drugs* in 1998 found: "Healthcare professionals have detected no indication of scrip-chasing or doctor-shopping among the patients for whom they have prescribed dronabinol." The same article found that the drug had a low potential for misuse and did not encourage users to pursue illegal drugs.

But what if nausea could be safely and securely addressed without needing to get a prescription from a doctor at all? What if CBD in particular could be an answer for patients who don't respond well to the drugs currently available?

In 2011, a study was published in the *British Journal of Psychopharmacology* titled "Cannabidiol, a non-psychotropic component of cannabis, attenuates vomiting and nausea-like behaviour via indirect agonism of 5-HT(1A) somatodendritic autoreceptors in the dorsal raphe nucleus." It sought to examine the possibility that CBD, though nonpsychoactive, could still act indirectly with the serotonin 5-HT1A receptor to treat nausea. The study involved testing the anti-nausea effects of CBD on lab animals (shrews) that had been made to feel sick to their stomachs in four different ways. What did the results of the research show?

CBD suppressed nicotine-, lithium chloride (LiCl)- and cisplatin 20mg·kg(-1), but not 40mg·kg(-1) induced vomiting in the S. murinus and LiCl-induced conditioned gaping in rats. Antiemetic and antinausea-like effects of CBD were suppressed by WAY100135 and the latter by WAY100635. When administered to the DRN: (i) WAY100635 reversed anti-nausea-like effects of systemic CBD, and (ii) CBD suppressed nausea-like effects, an effect that was reversed by systemic WAY100635. CBD also displayed significant potency (in a bell-shaped dose-response curve) at enhancing the ability of 8-OH-DPAT to stimulate [(35) S]GTPγS binding to rat brainstem membranes in vitro. Systemically administered CBD and 8-OH-DPAT synergistically suppressed LiCl-induced conditioned gaping. [. . .] These results suggest that CBD produced its anti-emetic/anti-nausea effects by indirect activation of the somatodendritic 5-HT(1A) autoreceptors in the DRN.

In layman's terms, the CBD successfully reduced three of the four kinds of nausea and did indeed do so by acting on the 5-HT1A receptors in the brain.

Two years later, the same journal published

another important animal study on CBD and nausea: "Cannabidiolic acid prevents vomiting in Suncus murinus and nausea-induced behaviour in rats by enhancing 5-HT1A receptor activation." This study looked at the effect of CBDA on nausea in rats and shrews. (CBDA is a sort of "precursor" to CBD. It is found in the raw form of cannabis. It is converted to CBD through decarboxylation when it is exposed to heat or sunlight.) The researchers here also chose to focus on anticipatory nausea—that is, the nausea you feel when you anticipate something unpleasant in your future. This kind of nausea is important for researchers to examine precisely because it does not have a clear-cut trigger that can be seen under a microscope. The study found that CBDA also worked *at least* as well as CBD on combating nausea, if not more so. Concluded the researchers: "CBDA shows promise as a treatment for nausea and vomiting, including anticipatory nausea for which no specific therapy is currently available."

In 2015, the journal *Psychopharmacology* published "Effect of selective inhibition of monoacylglycerol lipase (MAGL) on acute nausea, anticipatory nausea, and vomiting in rats and Suncus murinus." This study sought to examine the role of the endocannabinoid 2-arachodonyl glycerol (2-AG) on the regulation of nausea and vomiting. Researchers found that giving 2-AG to rats and shrews suppressed severe nausea and vomiting. Although it was not studying CBD—but instead a different endocannabinoid, 2-AG—the study was still important for our purposes because it again showed an endocannabinoid effectively fighting nausea.

Again, let me stress that I find testing on animals distasteful. However, the results published in these studies led to some truly exciting developments. More and more, scientists started to wonder if maybe the whole family of endocannabinoids could have anti-nausea properties.

Finally, in 2016, an article studying CBD's effect on nausea in humans—in addition to animals—was published in the journal *Cannabis and Cannabinoid Research*. Titled "Cannabinoid Regulation of Acute and Anticipatory Nausea," the study sought to examine the potential of CBD to treat the most serious nauseas that went untreated by other means. The study noted that the existing cannabis-based prescription drug Sativex® (which is not currently approved for use in the United States) has been shown reasonably effective at treating serious nausea but also pointed out that Sativex® is half-THC, half-CBD, and no researcher has yet shown if the anti-nausea effect is coming from the THC, the CBD, or both. By examining data from both animal models and studies on humans, the researchers were able to conclude that

The endocannabinoid system clearly plays an important role in the regulation of nausea. The pre-clinical findings suggest that CB1 receptor agonists, as well as FAAH and MAGL inhibitors, which elevate levels of AEA and 2-AG, respectively, reduce acute nausea and anticipatory nausea. As well, by a non cannabinoid mechanism of action, both CBD and CBDA are highly effective anti nausea treatments in these animal models without producing sedation or psychoactive effects. Nausea remains an elusive, difficult to control symptom in human chemotherapy patients and there are currently no selective treatments for anticipatory nausea. Clinical trials with FAAH inhibitors, MAGL inhibitors, CBD, and CBDA are warranted to improve the quality of life of patients undergoing cancer treatment by reducing the side effects of nausea and anticipatory nausea when it develops.

This was probably the most positive—and the most definitive—statement yet on the observable ability of CBD to help people who suffer from problems with stomach sickness and nausea.

There is more for us to learn about cannabinoids and nausea, and research is ongoing. THC, CBDA, and CBD all appear to be effective to different extents in making people feel less sick. I hope that in the future, new studies will help scientists to configure the perfect "cocktail" of the three that will help correct nausea most effectively.

Should you consider using CBD for the treatment of your nausea today? Well, because nausea without an obvious cause can sometimes be the sign of a more serious issue, you should see a physician first if you're feeling sick to your stomach but don't know why.

However, if you already know what is causing your nausea, then CBD might be right for you. For example, if you've tried other nausea medications that are *not* cannabinoid-based—and they haven't worked—then there is a real possibility that a treatment such as CBD could succeed where others have failed.

If you're dealing with temporary nausea from something harmless (but annoying) like motion-sickness or seasickness, it may be reasonable to try CBD as a first choice for treatment. Its antinausea effects have been observed scientifically, and it may be as effective (or even more effective) for you than something like dimenhydrinate (Dramamine). However, that study has yet to be done.

Nausea is something that affects everyone from time to time and impacts others to a very extreme degree. It's great that a wide selection of antinausea treatments and medications already exist. In this instance, we want to make sure that CBD augments existing therapies to get patients the best results possible. Anybody fighting a bad case of nausea needs all the help they can get—especially if the existing help isn't working so well. CBD can be a useful choice for physicians and patients to safely add to a nausea-treatment plan.

And if you're just dealing with occasional nausea from a well-understood origin, there's no reason you can't use CBD to fight it. Take some CBD in your favorite form and see if it provides you with some relief. The research shows there's a good chance it will work for you.

AUTISM SPECTRUM DISORDER

Autism is a developmental disorder that impacts tens of millions of people. It is not generally understood to be curable, but many people with autism respond to treatment and go on to have full and rewarding lives. Most diagnoses by pediatricians happen as young as two or three years old, and over the past decade medical professionals are increasingly well versed on the signs of autism. However, for many years it was often misdiagnosed as intellectual disability, schizophrenia, or even "mental retardation." Today, autism can be treated with a variety of medications and therapies (such as speech therapy and/or behavioral therapy). It is hard to understand trends in autism, since increased diagnoses may not stem from increased prevalence, but simply from better-informed physicians making more accurate diagnoses. In developed nations like the United States, over 1 percent of all children are diagnosed as autistic, and for unknown reasons about 80 percent of autism diagnoses occur in boys.

While many people with autism have controlled symptoms that allow them to lead essentially normal lives, the disorder generally causes impairments in social interaction, communication, restricted interests, and repetitive behavior. In this section, it is important for me to note that although I am presenting autism alongside medical conditions like asthma and migraines, there are many in the autism community who are passionate about viewing autism as a "different way of being" and not a disorder or disease. I want to be clear here that I am not saying that autism needs to be "cured" or "corrected" (with CBD or with anything else), but I think evidence is showing that people with autism can respond in positive ways to CBD, and my purpose here is to educate readers about those ways.

The causes of autism are still being studied. However, generally accepted medical wisdom holds that autism can run in families and be passed down genetically. It also seems to occur at a higher incidence in children whose mothers have abused alcohol and/or cocaine. Environmental factors, like exposure to pesticides and certain autoimmune diseases, may also play a role.

Both autism and CBD have seen a rise in clinical study in the twenty-first century, and in just the last few years several important research articles have been published hinting at the potential for people with autism to experience successful results from CBD.

In 2017, a team of researchers published "The Endocannabinoid System and Autism Spectrum Disorders: Insights from Animal Models" in the *International Journal of Molecular Sciences*. While only an animal study—about which, again, I have moral qualms—it suggested powerfully that the endocannabinoid system may be key for getting positive results for people with autism. The researchers experimented on mice that had been bred to exhibit "hyperactivity, repetitive behaviors, anxiety-related phenotypes, altered social behaviors" and other traits commonly associated with autistics. The animals were then treated with a wide variety of compounds designed to modulate the endocannabinoid system. The results? The researchers found that different stimulations impacted the symptoms of the mice to varying degrees. Though it was a very preliminary study—and very general when it came to how the endocannabinoid system was simulated—the researchers set out to prove what they hoped to prove, namely, that the endocannabinoid system *could* be used to impact the symptoms associated with autism. This meant that cannabinoids like CBD could be one of the keys for developing tools to help people with autism. As the researchers noted in their conclusion: "pharmacological interventions aimed at modulating the EC system could be beneficial for relieving symptoms associated with ASD [autism spectrum disorder]."

Also in 2017, another study laid more of the groundwork for cannabinoids to be tested as a good solution for autism. In the *Journal of Clinical Diagnostic Research*, a group of researchers from Saudi Arabia published "Role of Endocannabinoids on Neuroinflammation in Autism Spectrum Disorder Prevention." Drawing on cannabinoids' well-known ability to control inflammation, the Saudi researchers sought to examine if the anti-inflammatory effects might prove helpful for those with autism. To make their case, they examined the results of postmortem studies on people with autism and found that evidence of neuroinflammation—the inflammation of nervous tissue in the brain—was commonly observed. The Saudi team also found that "different proinflammatory cytokines such as, IL-1β, IL-6, IL-8, IL-12p40, and chemokines CCL2, CCL5, are elevated in ASD and are associated with poor communication and social interaction." The researchers concluded that it was reasonable to believe that the anti-inflammatory properties of cannabinoids would be likely to act on the parts of the brain that, when inflamed, could result in these symptoms. Further research found that this was indeed the case. Quoting the researchers: "in experimental models of AD, stimulation of CB1, CB2 and other non-CB1 and non-CB2 receptors with cannabinoids reduced microglial activation and microglia-mediated neurodegeneration." This means that the areas of the brain acted on by cannabinoids could act directly on these and other symptoms. The researchers found these results highly promising, believing a treatment that worked like CBD and other cannabinoids to act on these receptors in the brain could lessen or eliminate the inflammation associated with some symptoms of autism. As they put it in their conclusion:

This therapeutic use of drugs targeting EC system in CNS disorders has a great potential and animal experiments have shown encouraging results in reducing clinical symptoms in degenerative and inflammatory disease conditions. [. . .] The expected benefit from a chronic treatment aimed at stimulating the endocannabinoid system is a delayed progression of ASD: i.e., reduced inflammation, sustained potential for neurogenesis, and delayed memory impairment. Such results could lead to new therapeutic strategies that target the inflammation and the decline in neurogenesis associated ASD.

And during this year, another major study has provided heartening evidence of the ability of cannabinoids to help those with autism.

Earlier this year, a team of researchers from Israel writing in *Frontiers in Pharmacology* published the results of a trailblazing study: "Oral Cannabidiol Use in Children With Autism Spectrum Disorder to Treat Related Symptoms and Comorbidities." For many in the medical and autism communities, this was what they had been waiting for—a large-scale human trial of how CBD taken orally could help children with autism. And I do not exaggerate when I say the results were stunning. The children in the test (with an average age of eleven) were given CBD as oral drops, and their autism symptoms were monitored over several weeks. The Israeli researchers saw breathtaking improvements in many symptoms of autism in their test subjects. To list only some, 67.6 percent of subjects saw a lessening or elimination in rage attacks, violence toward others, and/or self-harm; 68.4 percent saw a lessening of hyperactivity and related behavior; a whopping 71.4 percent saw

an improvement in their sleep; and 47.1 percent experienced an improvement in anxiety, feeling less nervous and frightened. The study is still only a few months in but is already sending shockwaves across the CBD and autism communities. Here at last seems to be good proof that giving CBD to children with autism—in the kind of oral dosing a parent could easily administer and monitor—leads to good results controlling some of autism's most challenging symptoms. The researchers themselves also seemed convinced. The only call for further investigation in their paper was to say, "the long-term effects [of CBD on children] should be evaluated in large-scale studies."

In an age when clinical research can proceed at a pace that often feels frustratingly slow, autism has been a great exception to that rule. In just a few short years, research moved from beginning to prove that the ECS could be a pathway for accessing parts of the brain linked to autism symptoms to definitively showing that CBD tends to inhibit autism symptoms in children. If only research in all medical conditions related to CBD could move so quickly!

If you are an adult with autism looking for better symptom control, there is good reason to believe that an oral dose of CBD taken regularly may provide significant relief. (The Israeli study included no one older than twenty-two, but I suspect that what worked for children will also work for adults.) If you are the parent of a child with autism, I strongly encourage you to explore CBD-based treatment options with your child's physician. If the doctors who treat your child are not familiar with CBD research, you may need to educate them. (Steering them to the 2019 Israeli study is a good place to start!) In the years ahead, I think it's likely that CBD will emerge as one of the most common over-the-counter treatments for autism symptoms, because it's so effective and safe.

When it comes to autism and CBD, the research has been done; all that's left is for us to spread the good word!

OBESITY

Obesity is a national problem, and it's clear that there are numerous causes behind it. Larger food portions, a more sedentary lifestyle, a lack of access to fresh, healthy food in urban areas, and a whole panoply of other issues have created an incredible strain on our healthcare system as it struggles to deal with heavier and heavier Americans. We also know that obesity can often be a cause of other related medical conditions. If left untreated, it can shorten lives. For example, a 2014 study by the National Institutes of Health (NIH) found that extreme obesity (defined as a BMI—or Body Mass Index—of 40 or higher) had a reduction in lifespan equal to or higher than that of regular cigarette smokers.

Now, CBD isn't going to build new supermarkets in low-income neighborhoods, but there is evidence that it may be able to play a role in helping some maintain a healthy weight. Indeed, there is science to support it.

For a number of years, scientists and others have wondered if CBD might hold some of the keys to helping Americans lose weight. However, many found the notion counterintuitive because of the history of cannabis—specifically, stereotypes involving its causing "the munchies" and users often finding themselves in need of a snack. Yet while this "munchies effect" may be true in the short term, recent science has also established something surprising, namely, that people who use cannabis tend to weigh less than those who don't.

The 2011 study "Obesity and cannabis use: results from two representative national surveys" was published by researchers from Canada and involved data on over 50,000 people. The researchers found that people who used cannabis at least three days per week had a 14.3–17.2 percent chance of being obese, whereas the population that did not use cannabis had a 22–25.3 percent chance of being obese.

Something is obviously going on here that transcends munchies.

More and more, scientists think the action at play might not be the appetite-stimulating THC in cannabis, but instead the CBD. Though the THC might give some cannabis users an appetite, the effects of the CBD are more than making up for it.

How is this happening? Well, turns out there are a number of things CBD could be doing to help regulate weight.

Scientists have found that, at certain concentrations, CBD will connect to a receptor site on CB1 and cause it to prevent that receptor from binding to THC. Well, what does that mean? It means that the cause of some genetic obesity may be connected to overactivation of CB1 by the cannabinoids occurring naturally in our bodies. If those natural cannabinoids are restored to normal levels, then their tendency to make certain people gain weight could be limited—or even eliminated. This won't help people who simply choose to overeat and never go to the gym, but those who suffer from a genetic propensity to be overweight could find themselves back on a level playing field with everyone else.

But that's not all! Other studies on CBD and obesity have found that the former may be able to help regulate our metabolism—whether or not we also have a genetic predisposition to weight gain.

The 2017 study "Cannabinoid Receptor Signaling in Central Regulation of Feeding Behavior: A Mini-Review" published in *Frontiers in Neuroscience* examined the potential of cannabinoids to impact our eating habits and weight regulation. The researchers behind the study looked at the way cannabinoids interact with the CB1 receptor and that receptor's role in regulating energy, hunger, and feeding. They concluded that using CBD to target CB1 might result in the ability to "develop safe pharmacological interventions for the treatment of obesity."

What's interesting is that other studies have also suggested that CBD could impact our ability to regulate our weight . . . by targeting CB2.

For example, a study by Polish researchers titled "Cannabidiol decreases body weight gain in rats: involvement of CB2 receptors" experimented with giving large amounts of CBD to rats and then monitoring how they gained weight. Specifically, the rats were given two very large doses of CBD every day for two weeks. The researchers found that "doses of CBD produced significant decrease in body weight gain" among the rats. They concluded that "the results suggest that CBD has the ability to alter body weight gain, possibly via the CB2 receptor. CB2 receptors may play a role in the regulation of body weight and the effects of CB2 specific ligands should be further investigated in studies of body weight regulation."

Yet another study involving weight gain, CBD, and rats—this one titled "Cannabinol and cannabidiol exert opposing effects on rat feeding patterns" and published in *Psychopharmacology*—looked at how much rats would eat when given CBD. In this one, the results were a bit strange. The researchers found that

Cannabinol induced a CB(1)R-mediated increase in appetitive behaviors via significant reductions in the latency to feed and increases in consummatory behaviors via increases in meal 1 size and duration. Cannabinol also significantly increased the intake during hour 1 and total chow consumed during the test. Conversely, cannabidiol significantly reduced total chow consumption over the test period. Cannabigerol administration induced no changes to feeding behavior.

At first, CBD seemed to temporarily increase the appetites of the rats. But then, over time, it significantly reduced the amount of food that the rats chose to eat. The researchers believed this was somewhat novel because they'd never before seen CBD act to increase appetite—even if it later reduced it. However, what was vitally important in both of these studies was that CBD was shown to interact with the brain chemistry that controls our ability to gain or lose weight, as well as how much we eat.

Whether CB1 or CB2—or both—hold the key for future research on obesity is something yet to be seen, but it is heartening to imagine a future in which dieticians are able to suggest a certain amount of CBD to assist overweight individuals in returning to a healthy weight. Anything we can do to help Americans fight back against the obesity epidemic will be important in the days ahead. If CBD might hold just part of the answer, we ought to give it a try. The fact that it has been shown not just to cause individuals to lose weight, but to eat less is certainly an important clue to what is going on.

Many of the weight loss drugs currently available for physicians to prescribe have, as their goal, the reduction of overall caloric intake. People who eat just a few hundred calories less per day can see big results on the scale and in their waistlines. If we can harness the power of CBD to help people make healthier food choices that involve eating less overall, then obese individuals ought to be able to make real headway in getting back to a healthy weight.

The last thing to know about CBD and weight is that cannabinoids may promote the browning of fat cells. Humans have two types of fat in their bodies: white and brown. White fat is what most people think of when they think of fat. It represents excess calories used to provide insulation and cushion your organs. Unfortunately, having a lot of white fat tends to correlate to chronic illnesses like heart disease and Type 2 diabetes. Cutting the amount of white fat in your body can be an important step on the road to improving your health.

Then, on the other side of things, there is brown fat. Brown fat is what we burn when we exercise. Physicians find that healthy people tend to have more brown fat and less white fat. Sleeping well and cold temperatures can convert white fat into brown fat, and this has been known for some time. Anything else that might help people have less white fat in their bodies and more brown fat would be good for overall health.

CBD, it appears, may also do just that.

The study "Cannabidiol promotes browning in 3T3-L1 adipocytes" was published in the journal *Molecular Cell Biochemistry* by researchers from Korea in 2016. The study investigated whether CBD could be used to "brown" fat cells and thereby help curb obesity. Turns out it could. The researchers isolated fat cells in test tubes and treated them with CBD. When they did so, they discovered that, indeed, the cells began to send out the genes and proteins that change white fat into brown fat. As the researchers concluded:

These data suggest possible roles for CBD in browning of white adipocytes, augmentation of lipolysis, thermogenesis, and reduction of lipogenesis. In conclusion, the current data suggest that CBD plays dual modulatory roles in the form of inducing the brown-like phenotype as well as promoting lipid metabolism. Thus, CBD may be explored as a potentially promising therapeutic agent for the prevention of obesity.

Turning white fat into brown fat would be an easy way to help people with existing fat get healthier and potentially extend their lives by warding off more serious health issues down the line.

As with virtually everything we've seen regarding CBD and its positive effects, it seems to come at the problem from a variety of angles and may treat the same condition or symptom in multiple ways. If CBD can make us lose weight, eat less, and turn dangerous fat into less dangerous fat, then it's a powerful tool in anybody's weight loss arsenal. We may be eating less because we are less anxious, experiencing less inflammation, or because certain neurons in our brains are being triggered. If you ask me, it's *all* good!

While we can all think of a few overweight people who use cannabis, we can probably think of more skinny people who do so. (And those overweight people might actually be *more* overweight if they did not use cannabis!) But anecdotal evidence aside, the scientific studies leave no doubt in my mind that it is the CBD in cannabis that has allowed users to stay on the skinnier side for so long. By drawing on CBD today to fight weight gain, we can combine ancient wisdom and cutting-edge science to give people who need it a great new way of managing their weight.

If you're trying to lose some weight and looking for something to give you a little "edge" during your next diet, CBD might very well do the trick.

HEART HEALTH

Heart health is a serious issue. Heart disease is a leading killer in our country. Medical innovations in cardiovascular health are happening every day, and the science involved in protecting and repairing the heart is excellently funded and growing ever stronger—and medical intervention is not always necessary. Research shows that even small changes and improvements to one's heart health—such as eating a healthy diet and exercising—can have big impacts on one's longevity and quality of life. CBD also shows potential to be one of the many elements that could bolster heart health and help people suffer from fewer heart-related conditions.

As I'm sure you know, the heart pumps blood throughout our body and is necessarily linked to all the systems that make the process possible. Heart health impacts numerous parts of our body—and numerous systems in our body—and vice versa. For many people, the first sign that a heart-related issue may be on the horizon is the onset of high blood pressure. According to the CDC, 33 percent of all adult Americans have high blood pressure. The CDC also says that while about 54 percent of people with high blood pressure have their condition under control, the remainder do not. High blood pressure was a contributing cause of death for 410,000 Americans in 2014, and it costs our country tens of billions of dollars each year in healthcare expenses.

The good news is that studies are beginning to show that CBD can be a safe and effective way to lower blood pressure with little to no side effects.

A 2017 study in *JCI Insight*—a journal published by The American Society for Clinical Investigation—titled "A single dose of cannabidiol reduces blood pressure in healthy volunteers in a randomized crossover study" took healthy male volunteers and gave them a 600mg dose of CBD—or a placebo—and monitored their cardiovascular function. Their overall resting blood pressure was then taken, and so was their blood pressure during "stress tests" designed to increase it. The researchers' findings were as stated:

> Our data show that a single dose of CBD reduces resting blood pressure and the blood pressure response to stress, particularly cold stress, and especially in the post-test periods. This may reflect the anxiolytic and analgesic effects of CBD, as well as any potential direct cardiovascular effects. CBD also affected cardiac parameters but without affecting cardiac output. Given the increasing use of CBD as a medicinal product, these hemodynamic changes should be considered for people taking CBD. Further research is also required to establish whether CBD has any role in the treatment of cardiovascular disorders such as hypertension.

In plain English, the CBD lowered the blood pressure of the people who took it. It also reduced the tendency of certain stressors to make blood pressure go up, with no other impact on the function of the heart. (Elsewhere in the study, it is also noted that there were no other side effects, period.) The researchers see opportunity for more studies in the future, and potentially for CBD's use as a vehicle for controlling blood pressure.

Other studies on CBD and the heart suggest that, in addition to lowering blood pressure, it may be able to "come at" the issue of heart health from novel directions and so augment any existing treatments.

For example, take "Cannabidiol attenuates cardiac dysfunction, oxidative stress, fibrosis, inflammatory and cell death signaling pathways in diabetic cardiomyopathy." This study from 2010 found that CBD can reduce inflammation and cell death, which are also associated with heart disease. Using rats as test subjects, the researchers in this study found that CBD reduced oxidative stress and prevented heart disease from occurring in the first place in the mice. What does this mean for humans potentially? Quoth the researchers:

> Collectively, these results coupled with the excellent safety and tolerability profile of cannabidiol

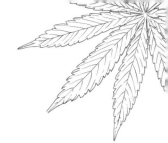

in humans, strongly suggest that it may have great therapeutic potential in the treatment of diabetic complications, and perhaps other cardiovascular disorders, by attenuating oxidative/nitrosative stress, inflammation, cell death and fibrosis.

So CBD can lower blood pressure *and* help keep damage to the heart from occurring in the first place? Sounds to me like we have another winner. As with many conditions we've reviewed, two things remain constant. First, more research needs to be done. (At the very least, I think tests should be conducted to see how CBD impacts people who are already on medications to help with heart function.) And second, we once again see the interrelation of the human body impacted by the wide variety of improvements to our health that CBD is known to make. Our hearts are impacted by obesity, stress, anxiety and worrying, high blood pressure, certain kinds of inflammation, and other triggers. The fact that CBD is known to touch upon all of these areas makes it easy to guess that the heart would also be positively affected.

If you have a serious heart condition—or you've been having serious symptoms—you absolutely need to be under the care of a physician. However, your heart doctor may encourage you to use CBD as a remedy, probably in concert with other treatments, as more research emerges. And given CBD's ability to lower blood pressure, those who take it regularly may delay the onset of their own heart troubles, possibly even preventing them.

GENERAL BRAIN HEALTH

We've looked at the heart, so what about the brain? Here too, remarkable work is being done to suggest that CBD may have powerful beneficial contributions to make. We've looked at epilepsy and psychosis, which are largely considered to be diseases of the brain. But there is also general brain health. Things like attentiveness, cognition, memory, and processing speed all impact people's daily lives, and all fall under the heading of brain function or brain health.

To begin looking at CBD's impact on the brain, we can review what has been established thus far regarding its interaction with neurotransmitters. Neurotransmitters are the go-betweens that allow brain calls to communicate with one another, passing signals from cell to cell as they move throughout the brain. Much of the work of neurotransmitters is done automatically, without being prompted by a conscious thought. Similar to smooth muscle—the automatic muscles that move food down the esophagus, for example—neurotransmitters are constantly working to ensure that things like breathing, swallowing, and digestion occur. When neurotransmitters run into problems or fall out of balance, it can be bad for everybody, so to speak. Things like stress and anxiety can impact neurotransmitters, but they can also be affected by environmental factors, personal genetics, and certain medications.

Scientists are beginning to understand

how and why CBD can bolster neurotransmitter function in the brain. But even before the hard science came copious anecdotal evidence from people who use CBD regularly. These users said that CBD helps them with thinking clearly and eliminates "brain fog." (There is, of course, no medical definition for brain fog—it is hardly a technical term—but generally when people use it, they are talking about a lack of mental clarity. It can also conjure difficulty recalling things, forgetfulness, difficulty focusing, difficulty recognizing things, and a generally thick-headed feeling.)

People who suffer from brain fog have found time and again that CBD seems to relieve their symptoms. They think more clearly, feel more alert, and seem to have better recall for things like names and faces. But what is really going on here? The symptoms of brain fog are, themselves, so difficult to pin down that some have thought the good effects produced by CBD might simply be psychosomatic. Is there any "there" there, when it comes to CBD and brain function?

This is what researchers are now discovering.

In 2017, the paper "An Update on Safety and Side Effects of Cannabidiol: A Review of Clinical Data and Relevant Animal Studies" was published in the journal *Cannabis and Cannabinoid Research*. This article noted that studies have established how CBD can be used to actually increase the levels of two kinds of neurotransmitters—serotonin and glutamate. Serotonin is extremely valuable for the parts of the brain that control personality and mood, and glutamate is key for learning, recognition, and memory. By increasing these types of neurotransmitters, researchers found that it was reasonable to conclude that CBD was boosting these positive mental traits in the subjects.

Another interesting study on CBD and overall brain function was published in 2019 in *Psychopharmacology*. The paper was titled "Effects of cannabidiol on brain excitation and inhibition systems: a randomised placebo-controlled single dose trial during magnetic resonance spectroscopy in adults with and without autism spectrum disorder." (If you are skipping around in this book, note that a previous section goes into greater detail on CBD and autism.) The study sought to discover the effects of CBD on the brain pathways that are thought to most affect people with autism. Subjects—some with autism, some without—took doses of CBD and had their brains scanned at regular intervals to look for changes. What the researchers found was very interesting. A large, single dose of CBD seemed to boost levels of neurotransmitter activity in people both with and without autism. Specifically, the researchers were interested in what they saw when it came to CBD's ability to boost a neurotransmitter called GABA that is known to impact impulses between nerve cells in the brain. Historically, GABA has been thought to impact anxiety and mood, as well as affect epilepsy and pain. Said the researchers:

The corollary of our observations is that because CBD 'shifts' glutamate and GABA+, it may affect glutamatergic excitation and GABAergic inhibition, and thereby impact on brain function. We did not directly test this here, but some support for this proposition comes from a recent report that CBD increases prefrontostriatal functional connectivity in neurotypical controls. However, our results predict that the direction of a functional response to CBD may be distinct in autistic individuals, and this warrants further investigation. [. . .] Additional studies will be required to (i) identify the neural basis of the response to acute CBD challenge, including potential pharmacologically homogeneous sub-groups within the autistic spectrum; (ii) examine potential functional consequences of CBD challenge in terms of inhibition, brain network activity, cognition, and behaviour; and (iii) investigate whether an acute response to CBD could predict the effects of sustained treatment in ASD.

As studies go, this was not the best one for showing that CBD could help people with autism (other CBD studies have done that better). However, while calling for more research, the authors made it clear that this was definitive proof that CBD had a positive effect on the neurotransmitters in human brains. While these researchers had been hoping for autism-related findings, what they ended up establishing may have been a much larger conclusion, namely, that CBD is able to impact the neurotransmitters that regulate some of the brain's most important excitation and inhibition systems, including those linked to overall brain health and function.

Do these early studies show definitively what is happening with CBD and the brain? Absolutely not. But we do know what CBD is doing. It is interacting with some of the neurotransmitters that can impact many aspects of thinking, mental clarity, and mental health. And it is boosting and bolstering them, not hindering them (at least not in any way that has yet been detected).

The effect of CBD on general brain health is likely to be one of the areas where our knowledge about CBD grows more slowly. This is because many of the discoveries will likely be made by researchers who are seeking information about a specific ailment or disease. Even so, we can now confidently say that we know brain health can be positively impacted by CBD.

If your experience is that CBD helps you think more clearly and achieve greater mental acuity—that's great. In addition to your personal experience, the science backs you up; CBD has positive effects on the neurotransmitters in our brain. Fully understanding—and fully harnessing—those beneficial effects will be the next exciting step.

In the meantime, if you'd like to see if taking CBD helps you think more clearly, I absolutely encourage you to give it a shot!

CANCER

Cancer. Just the world by itself conjures grief and terror.

Why would I choose cancer to end—rather than begin—this chapter on medical conditions?

Well, I do so because I firmly believe that the potential impact of CBD on cancer patients is poised to become the next revolution in this field. And if it is, the consequences will be truly world-shattering.

Cancer enacts a grievous toll on our society. Each year, 1.7 million Americans are diagnosed with cancer, and over 600,000 will die of the disease. Close to 40 percent of all Americans will be diagnosed with a form of cancer at some point in their lifetimes. According to the National Cancer Institute, the cost of caring for people with cancer in the United States is nearly $150 billion.

Almost everyone knows someone whose life has been significantly impacted by cancer. It brings with it anxiety, fear, and often tremendous pain. Even a small reduction in pain and suffering for cancer patients is worth pursuing. Furthermore, as cancer impacts so many people and is one of the leading causes of death for Americans, it is poised to be one of the most important subsets in the field of CBD studies.

The connections between CBD and cancer start with the connections between cannabis and cancer. Prior to the twenty-first century, there were many anecdotal cases of folks using cannabis to relieve pain related to cancer. People who had serious pain because of cancer treatments—or had end-stage pain—sometimes found that smoking marijuana could help them better manage their pain.

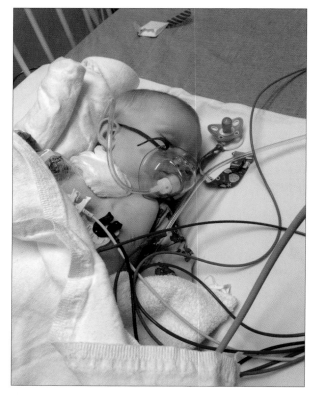

Sophie, prepped for surgery.

But what was the effect on their health? There, there was more controversy.

Were people shortening their lives by using cannabis? Could it hasten the advance of their cancers, or give healthy people cancer in the first place?

Some people wondered if Americans who used cannabis by smoking "marijuana cigarettes" were taking the same health risks as those who smoked tobacco regularly.

However, in the 1990s, a landmark study by the Kaiser Permanente Medical Care Program of nearly 65,000 people—including regular and occasional smokers of cannabis—found that regular smokers of marijuana did not face the same smoking-related health risks as regular tobacco smokers. There was possible evidence that smoking marijuana, but not tobacco, could be linked to an increased risk of prostate cancer in men, and cervical cancer in women. The same study found that cannabis users had a 45 percent lower chance of developing bladder cancer. While scientists have long known that marijuana smoke can produce carcinogens, they are not identical to the carcinogens found in cigarette smoke. Even today, the links between inhaled marijuana smoke and cancer remain inconclusive.

Though it is derived from hemp, taking CBD does not expose the human body to any of the carcinogens present in marijuana smoke. There is no evidence that anyone who already has cancer could see their cancer progress more quickly if they take CBD.

Most of the scientists and researchers who have begun to experiment at the intersection of CBD and cancer have done so in the subfield of cancer-related pain.

When it comes to controlling cancer pain, the leading researchers have tended to concentrate on the intersection of CBD and THC, and how the pair can be used in tandem to control cancer-related pain.

One important study in this connection was published in 2010 in the *Journal of Pain and Symptom Management* and was titled "Multicenter, Double-Blind, Randomized, Placebo-Controlled, Parallel-Group Study of the Efficacy, Safety, and Tolerability

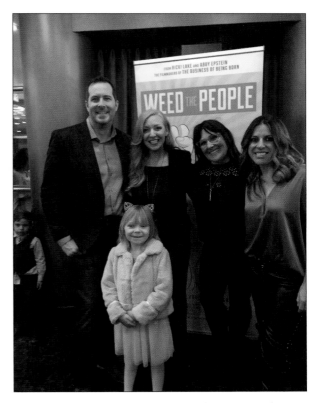

Sophie and family with Ricki Lake, featured at the *Weed the People* event.

of THC:CBD Extract and THC Extract in Patients with Intractable Cancer-Related Pain." The study compared the effects of a combination of THC and CBD, of THC alone, and of a placebo on relieving pain in patients with advanced cancer. These patients still suffered pain despite heavy application of opioid painkillers. Nearly 180 patients participated in the study. The results show that the combination of CBD and THC—more than THC alone—had the greatest and most effective reduction in patient pain. According to the rating scale used, patient pain was reduced

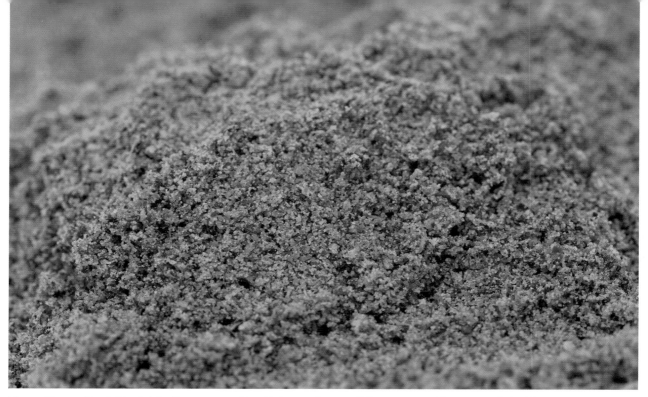

Hemp Flower (buds) is rich in Omegas, making it the perfect additive to smoothies or medicinal beverages.

by about 30 percent. Most remarkably, the patients who took only THC had a pain reduction score that was close to the group taking the placebo. *Something special is going on with CBD*, thought these researchers. They concluded that a THC and CBD extract is effective and recommended for alleviating pain in cancer patients whose pain is not fully eliminated by opioids.

A few years later, in 2013, another important study in the same journal built on this work. The study, "An Open-Label Extension Study to Investigate the Long-Term Safety and Tolerability of THC/CBD Oromucosal Spray and Oromucosal THC Spray in Patients With Terminal Cancer-Related Pain Refractory to Strong Opioid Analgesics," delved into attempting to treat the serious pain of end-stage cancer patients with a THC–CBD spray over a longer period of time. These patients were being given extremely high doses of opioid painkillers, and still their pain was not relieved. Building on the work of previous studies, which showed this as an effective way of treating cancer pain, this study aimed to test the tolerability of this method of pain treatment in the demographic that probably needed it most. As in the above study, patients were given a spray that contained a THC–CBD mix, just THC, or a placebo. The patients were allowed to self-administer the spray to alleviate the pain. When the study was completed, once again, it was the THC–CBD combination spray that had the best results, helping several of the patients who used it to lower their pain ranking score and decrease their pain. In addition, the study found no side effects or related health concerns from the spray. And perhaps most important, the spray showed no loss of effect over time for the patients who were using it. They did not "adjust to it" and/or require higher doses as time went by. Once again, we saw CBD as an integral component of a potentially valuable solution for easing cancer pain.

However, not all researchers have looked solely into CBD as pain control for cancer.

In 2016, a group of Polish researchers from Jagiellonian University Medical College published an academic paper titled "Cannabinoids—a new weapon against cancer?" In it, they reported that experiments carried out on cell lines and initial testing have shown that phytocannabinoids, endocannabinoids, and synthetic cannabinoids can arrest the growth of many types of tumors and prevented tumors from metastasizing. These researchers concluded that it then follows that research on cannabinoids might logically yield a tool for the fight against cancer.

A 2019 study, also by researchers from Eastern Europe and published in the *International Journal of Molecular Sciences*, titled "Future Aspects for Cannabinoids in Breast Cancer Therapy," seemed to bridge the gap between pain and treatment. The paper begins by examining the existing evidence that cannabinoids can "provide relief for tumor-associated symptoms (including nausea, anorexia, and neuropathic pain) in the palliative treatment of cancer patients." They also found that "Additionally, they may decelerate tumor progression in breast cancer patients." The

researchers note the ability of CBD and THC to impact "tumor aggressiveness" in breast cancers. Most of the research in this study came from animal test models, and as the researchers themselves noted in the paper: "at present, clinical trials . . . in [human] cancer patients are rare." However, because "CBD and THC, exhibit beneficial anti-inflammatory or antitumoral properties . . . [they are] promising agents for inhibiting breast cancer progression." The researchers conclude by pointing out that cannabinoids are already given to women in the later stages of breast cancer—with an eye to quelling pain—and it might be no great leap for future researchers to begin testing cannabinoids at earlier stages of cancer to test their ability "to decelerate tumor progression."

We live at a time in history when remarkable innovations in cancer care and research are making such breakthroughs possible. I started this section by noting some of the troubling statistics about the toll of cancer on Americans today, but there are also some encouraging statistics to share. According to the National Cancer Institute—because of breakthroughs in treatment—the overall cancer death rate in the US fell by 26 percent between 1991 and 2015! This means that the number of cancer survivors has also increased. Yet this also potentially means that the number of cancer survivors—some of whom also must deal with cancer-related pain—has increased as well.

What the future holds for cancer in the United States is not completely known.

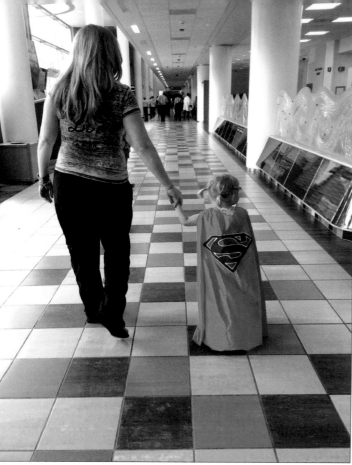

Sophie Supergirl taking a stroll with her Supermom, Tracy Ryan.

Continued scientific and medical innovations may push the death rate from cancer lower still in the years ahead. On the other hand, the nation's obesity epidemic shows no sign of stopping, and the Baby Boomers are continuing to age. Obesity and advanced age are both risk factors for cancer. Clearly, we have our work cut out for us.

I want CBD to be part of the solution—both for pain control, and for looking at ways we can stop people from contracting cancer in the first place.

I saved cancer for the final disease in this section because I believe that it may hold the pathway—literally—for the increased public understanding and acceptance of CBD. When something demonstrates an ability to fight cancer (or stop cancer pain), society has a way of getting behind it. This seems to cross every part of our culture, every religion, and every party line. In 1971, President Richard Nixon famously declared a "War on Cancer" and asked congress for $100 million (over $600 million in today's dollars) in new funds for cancer research. The request was granted . . . and then some! By the time it was finished, the National Cancer Act of 1971 had created the National Cancer Institute and given it an annual budget of $400 million. Members of congress from both sides of the aisle voted for it—confident that such a vote would not be politically risky. If anything, a vote to fight cancer made politicians stronger. In his speech about the

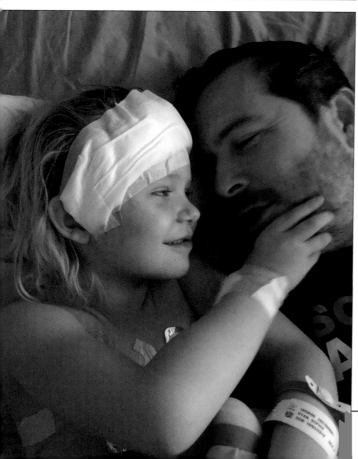

Sophie and her Dad snuggling after surgery.

campaign, Nixon said: "Let us make a total national commitment to achieve this goal." The country seemed ready to do just that.

In the years since, Americans have incorporated new foods into their diets, adopted new health-screening habits, and cut down drastically on cigarette smoking—all with an eye to preventing cancer. Stopping cancer has become something of a national rallying cry, and for good reason. Today, the National Cancer Institute's budget is nearly $6 billion per year. Cancer research constitutes nearly 9 percent of the National Institutes of Health's total annual budget. But it goes beyond government work. The American Cancer Society now receives approximately three-quarters of a billion dollars in private donations from Americans each year.

I firmly believe that if CBD can become a powerful tool in the arsenal for preventing and treating cancer, then Americans across all parts of our culture—across all demographics—will drop any stigma about CBD that they ever may have had. If our nation's governmental and personal funding of cancer research is any indication, then Americans will all but *demand* that more research studies be green-lit to harness CBD's healing properties.

Once CBD has entered the public consciousness as an accepted cancer fighter, it will be commonplace to see it used to treat other conditions—from the mild to the serious. There may, perhaps, be no more important outcome than to see CBD used as a cancer-fighting drug. Millions and millions of people stand to be helped in profound ways. It is simply a win-win. Nothing in the world of CBD gets me more excited.

I hope it also gets you excited!

THE ENTOURAGE EFFECT

As a final note, a term you may encounter when researching the health effects of CBD is "the Entourage Effect." What does it mean, and why is it so named?

Technically, "entourage" is the name for a group of people who surround an important person, usually providing some type of assistance. (Think of the entourage that follows around a pop star or Hollywood actor.) Sometimes the term "entourage effect" has been used in cuisine to describe ingredients acting together to flavor a food or make a meal more nutritious. However, when it comes to the world of CBD, you'll see that the term is being used to describe a powerful natural phenomenon that suggests that the active ingredients in cannabis act together to have a healthful effect bigger than the sum of their parts. Like an entourage, the cannabinoids work together—and with other natural substances—to help each component do more.

The most common example of the entourage effect is usually the interaction between CBD and THC. In studies where participants tested the abilities of CBD, THC, and CBD–THC to address their ailment or cure their pain, in almost every case the CBD–THC was most effective, and *this combined version is also more effective than the results from CBD-alone added to THC-alone.* Something about CBD and THC together is special. When used at the same time, the effects that they have are boosted. (One clue that it's the organic cannabinoids at play in this "entourage" is that the combined benefit is not present when CBD is combined with synthetic THC.) Researchers now think that cultivars could be created to take advantage of these qualities.

The idea that cannabis could be "tuned" so that its active compounds "help" one another to increase their effects is a powerful idea. Is there any clinical evidence to support it? As it turns out, there is.

When applied to cannabinoids, most people believe that the first use of the term "entourage effect" arose from a 1999 study titled "An entourage effect: inactive endogenous fatty acid glycerol esters enhance 2-arachidonoyl-glycerol cannabinoid activity, published in the European Journal of Pharmacology." In this study—by numerous authors, including Raphael Mechoulam—the research team reported on findings that showed how cannabinoid receptors were impacted by different chemical components, and also that some cannabinoids used together in related systems could boost one another's impact. In short, the researchers had found that the cannabinoids in cannabis and hemp tended to work together with other chemicals naturally occurring in those plants to produce a better overall outcome for users.

It was a bold claim, but subsequent researchers were intrigued and continued looking into the possibility of the effect. In 2011, the *British Journal of Pharmacology* published "Taming THC: potential cannabis synergy and phytocannabinoid-terpenoid entourage effects" by Ethan B. Russo. This article reviewed the "echelon of phytotherapeutic agents, the cannabis terpenoids: limonene, myrcene, α-pinene, linalool, β-caryophyllene, caryophyl-

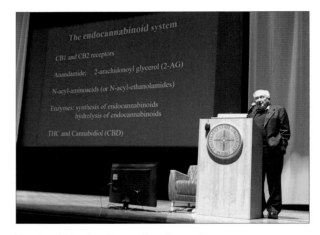

Raphael Mechoulam talks about the endocannabinoid system within all mammals and how receptors in our body perceive cannabinoids.

lene oxide, nerolidol and phytol" believed to play a role in the effect. Specifically, the author looked to discover "phytocannabinoid-terpenoid interactions that could produce synergy with respect to treatment of pain, inflammation, depression, anxiety, addiction, epilepsy, cancer, fungal and bacterial infections."

Not only did the researcher find that, indeed, these elements did interact together to boost their respective effects, but that their boosted effects might be particularly useful in medicine for treating "treatment-resistant depression, anxiety, drug dependency, dementia and a panoply of dermatological disorders." And in his conclusion, the author noted:

> . . . that selective breeding of cannabis chemotypes rich in ameliorative phytocannabinoid and terpenoid content offer complementary pharmacological activities that may strengthen and broaden clinical applications and improve the therapeutic index of cannabis extracts containing THC, or other base phytocannabinoids. Psychopharmacological and dermatological indications show the greatest promise.

Not only was the entourage effect real, but it was something that could be manipulated and enhanced through selective breeding of cannabis and hemp plants.

The most recent research into the entourage effect can be found in "Cannabis, from plant to pill," published in the *British Journal of Clinical Pharmacology* late last year. The research in this article further explored the means by which cannabinoids can contribute synergistically to one another's positive effects and also examined how cultivation of cannabis varieties could become a tool for harnessing these effects. The author finds tremendous potential in cultivating cannabis and hemp that harnesses the entourage effect and creates "greater medical efficacy" for the plants involved. He also notes that because evidence for the effect is mostly anecdotal and on a case-by-case basis, large-scale double-blind clinical trials ought to be conducted for confirmation.

From these three major scientific articles, it seems to me that there's good reason to believe that the entourage effect exists, and that we may only be seeing the beginning of its uses. CBD and its health effects are already so powerful; the idea that there might be a way to unlock *even more* healthful properties by tuning its interaction with other cannabinoids is very exciting. It may be the next great leap forward in CBD.

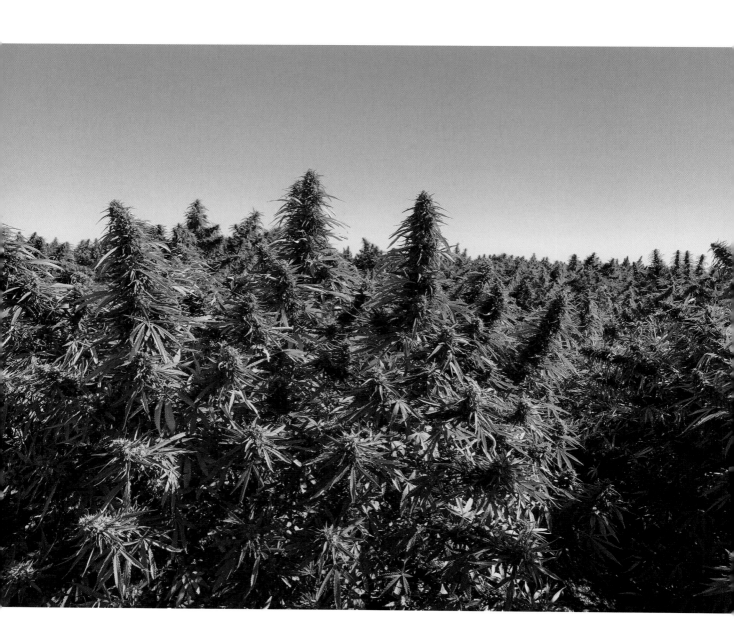

CHAPTER THREE
CBD VISIONARIES AT THE LEADING EDGE

Revolutions come about for many reasons. In science and technology, they often arise because of paradigm shifts. These shifts allow us to see things we never noticed before, or to see old things in an entirely new way.

The earliest advances in CBD came from cannabis research. The initial breakthrough—or, I should say, *one* of the initial breakthroughs of early research—resulted in a paradigm shift in both the scientific community and the general population. Put plainly, the breakthrough involved establishing that cannabis is not "one thing" but "many things." That is, many different compounds working in tandem.

Early research going back thirty years (and more) involved scientists teasing apart the various compounds in cannabis that produced different effects for users. This seems so obvious and self-evident to us today that it is hard to emphasize just how groundbreaking it was back in the day.

In the 2010s, a new generation of CBD researchers emerged to carry the torch forward. These remarkable physicians and scientists are leading the way by steering the focus of CBD in revolutionary new directions while making the breakthroughs that will change people's lives.

There are many young people who are choosing to make a career researching the impacts of CBD. If you're a young person interested in health and science—and who wants to be at the forefront of making the world a better place—I'd like to encourage you to consider CBD. Some of the finest minds and the most entrepreneurial spirits are choosing to make a career researching the effects of CBD. From my experience, it's only once a generation that a true "greenfield" in new research opens up for scientists to pursue. That's what's happening now in CBD. Because of the wide variety of areas where CBD makes a positive impact, it is hard to find an area of focus within medicine where it *doesn't* have potential applications.

I'm also personally proud of the people in this chapter, as they were researching CBD—in many cases, staking their careers on it—when

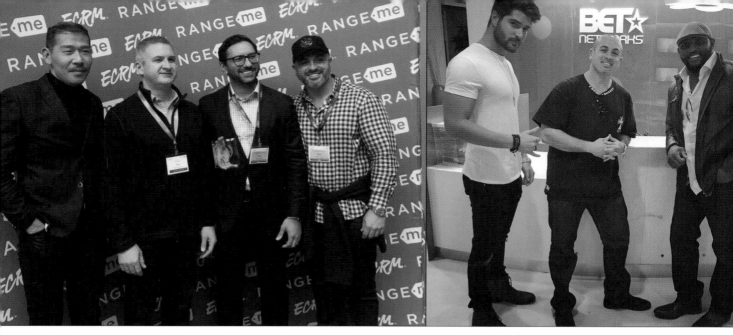

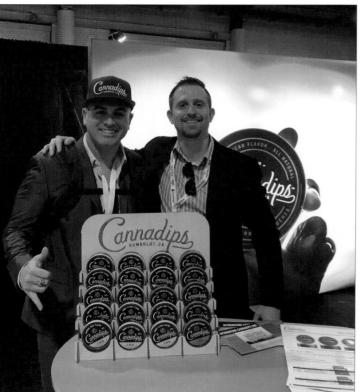

TOP: At ECRM 2019 in Chicago receiving an award for the most innovative CBD product. BOTTOM: Ryan Lewis with friend and founder of CannaDips, Case Mandel, who created the first cannabis-infused smokeless pouches.

it was still very much a dangerous thing to do. These researchers took a tremendous professional risk. They knew that their work meant that they would be incorrectly associated with recreational marijuana use. They knew that they were studying a substance that many felt was "too good to be true" and couldn't possibly deliver the results that were being claimed. They would risk being looked down upon by colleagues and entirely misunderstood by the public. They elected to start down the path of CBD research well before the "CBD boom," when success and financial reward were far from assured.

And they did not care.

They dedicated their careers to harnessing the positive, healing traits of CBD because it was the right thing to do. They were unconcerned about social stigma. They were willing to take the risk—putting their own careers and livelihoods at stake—because they had an early inkling of the extent to which CBD could help people. And they realized that if they were correct, if they could actually harness this power, then it would allow them to do incredibly meaningful work for the rest of their lives.

I'm so glad that these researchers chose to be brave. As you read about them here, I think you're going to be glad, too.

As I've found with my own focus on entrepreneurship and helping people, some things in life are a calling. There is work that some people are simply meant to do. These scientists and physicians have been called to work in CBD.

After you read their stories, maybe you will find that you have the same calling.

DR. ETHAN RUSSO

Dr. Ethan Russo is an MD with a degree from the University of Massachusetts Medical School. His work is on the cutting edge of developing medical approaches using hemp cannabinoids like CBD for activation of the human endocannabinoid system—or "ECS"—to treat symptoms that hinder the quality of life.

Russo has a strong background in clinical trials, and the experience necessary when trying to bring a new, safe drug or supplement to market. He also has a strong interest in medicinal plants—of all varieties—which he incorporates into both his medical practice and scientific research. He also has a background in neurology and pediatric neurology, which is very appropriate, as these are two of the areas where some of the most exciting CBD study is underway.

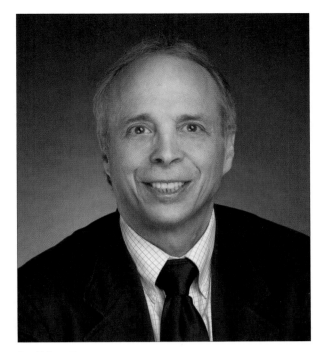

Dr. Ethan Russo

One of the reasons I like Dr. Russo so much is that he is willing to go wherever he needs, and meet with anybody, to get things done. He has studied in the Amazon rainforest in Peru, analyzing the native medicinal plants of the Machiguenga. He has also been a leading advocate for scientists fighting to gain approval from the US government to study cannabis. When cannabis became legal for medical purposes in California in 1996, he spent four years lobbying the FDA for approval to study its impact on people with migraines.

Today, a part of Dr. Russo's focus is in the gastrointestinal functions and, more specifically, the function of gut microbes and how they relate to homeostasis in humans. In an article published in 2016 covering gut bacteria biodiversity, he addresses the importance of the human endocannabinoid system (ECS) and that a clinical deficiency, or inactivation of the ECS, results in many of the gastrointestinal/inflammation issues we face today including but not limited to irritable bowel syndrome, chronic migraines, and fibromyalgia.

His company—Phytechs—is doing important work showing how modulating the ECS can have a positive effect on a staggering number of conditions and diseases. Because the ECS is one of the largest homeostatic systems in the human body—impacting the brain and every other major organ—Dr. Russo believes that as researchers learn to modulate the ECS using CBD, they will unlock an entirely new chapter in disease prevention, care, and treatment. We all have neural networks in our brains that communicate with other parts of our body through electrical impulses, and these impulses drive the release of neurotransmitters into synapse. Dr. Russo and his team believe that this action is key to understanding and harnessing the power of CBD. Endocannabinoid signaling is very important through the brain and spinal cord, and his research is making clear the extent to which CBD can impact it.

Specifically, Dr. Russo is interested in how CBD holds the potential to benefit sufferers of Parkinson's disease (PD) and Alzheimer's disease (AD). As he told *Forbes* magazine in an interview in early 2019, research in this area is also beginning to bear fruit:

> In a mouse model of PD, treatment with nabiximols (Sativex®), a cannabis-based pharmaceutical approved in 30 countries outside the USA, resulted

in improvement in dopamine neurotransmitter function, and reduced oxidative stress (akin to "rust" of the nervous system), as well as leading to improvements in anxiety and self-injury behaviors.

Clinical results with treatment of PD with cannabis have been quite mixed. Cannabidiol (CBD) helped a few PD patients with psychotic symptoms, and some with a rapid-eye movement sleep disorder. Observational studies with smoked cannabis, presumably high in THC, reportedly produced acute benefits on tremor, rigidity and slow movement (bradykinesia). The best results in PD were reported in a Czech study in 2004, in which patients ate raw leaves of cannabis for as much as three months and reported significant improvement in overall function, tremor, bradykinesia and rigidity, with few side effects.

[…]

The story in AD is even more intriguing. Both THC and CBD have been shown to interfere with the production of abnormal toxic matter in the brain of such patients. This is quite exciting, inasmuch as synthetic drugs designed for similar purposes have yet to advance in the clinic. Both THC and particularly CBD are known neuroprotective agents that hold the potential to slow or perhaps even halt the degenerative process. On the symptom side, THC as a single agent has proven beneficial in AD patients in reducing nocturnal agitation, improving sleep and appetite. Observations of nursing home patients in California with dementia have produced similar benefits as well as reducing the need for nursing intervention and amounts of other drugs.

There are four FDA-approved pharmaceuticals to treat memory loss in AD, but all have mild benefits on a temporary basis. These are designed to increase the amount of acetylcholine, the memory molecule in the brain that becomes depleted in AD. Interestingly, the terpenoid alpha-pinene is capable of boosting acetylcholine by inhibiting its breakdown, and with fewer side effects than the conventional drugs.

Dr. Russo's expertise in both CBD *and* THC allows him to speak definitively when he is interviewed by the press. He does not shrink away from mentioning THC and can be trusted to give an honest accounting of the progress he has seen. In the *Forbes* interview, he was able to lay out the benefits that researchers are beginning to see, but without exaggerating or sugarcoating the results.

I also like Dr. Russo because he is not shy about calling it like he sees it when it comes to the bad rep that CBD has gotten. Whenever interviewed, he makes it clear that he is not a prohibitionist and that he sees the slow progress on CBD today as an unfortunate by-product of this tendency toward THC prohibition. He also—like some other CBD researchers—does not hesitate to say that the dangers of THC have been greatly exaggerated by various groups including both media and politicians. When examining some treatments and studies, Dr. Russo has occasionally concluded that a CBD compound functions more effectively when THC is also present (in more than trace amounts). On these occasions, he does not hesitate to say that treatments with larger amounts of THC should be pursued.

Another reason that Dr. Russo is so respected—by me and many others—is that he's legitimately interested in improving the overall health of patients, and he knows that CBD- and THC-based treatments are only one step in the process. He is deeply interested in how probiotics and prebiotics can impact our gut bacteria and change our overall well-being. In addition to CBD, when he is interviewed, he also notes that vigorous exercise and anti-inflammatory diets—like the Mediterranean diet, heavy in fish and olive oils—have the potential to contribute to a healthy, pain-free life in the same areas that CBD does. In short, he never characterizes CBD as a one-and-done cure-all. Rather, he advocates for its place in a pantheon of healthy habits that can allow us to live longer, fuller, healthier lives.

Dr. Russo has done some of the most important work into the potential for the interaction of CBD with other drugs. It's important that Dr. Russo has been such a dedicated leader in this space, because it's probably the number one thing that people are concerned about. He is also keen to share his findings—which have been minimal. Dr. Russo has only found negative drug interactions with CBD when it is given in extremely high amounts, and even in these cases the side effects are rare.

Dr. Russo is a well-respected and educated medical professional with more than a decade of his life dedicated to GW Pharmaceuticals, where he became interested in fighting the opioid crisis with hemp. An interview published in 2017 discussed the very real potential hemp has with chronic pain sufferers and that a decrease in traditional pain relief management methods with drugs, like Hyrdocodone, would prevent many harmful side effects and the severe addiction potential that comes with opioid use. He has made clear that, like me, he is driven by the stark need to provide an alternative to addictive opioids when it comes to managing serious pain. For example, in a January 2019 interview with *Project CBD*, Dr. Russo noted the following:

> This is an absolute medical crisis in that 72,000 Americans died of opioid-related overdoses in 2017. We have known — and this may come as a surprise to almost everyone — it's been known for 150 years that cannabis is capable of acting in concert with opioids to treat pain and allowing what's called "opioid sparing." This means a lower dose producing the same or better level of pain control. Additionally, it was observed in the 19th century that cannabis could treat withdrawal symptoms from opioids and other addictive drugs, reduce craving, and allow people to get off of them entirely. The same thing has been observed for decades in people who have used cannabis medicinally. But, again, until recently that was primarily with THC predominant cannabis, which did work in this regard. But the real missing ingredient until say the last decade has been cannabidiol. Because cannabidiol on its own acts as an anti-addictive substance. It actually works on an area of the brain called the insula that reduces craving. Particularly in combination with THC, we've seen a really amazing response in patients to reduce their opioid doses and often get off of opioids that they may have used chronically. Additionally, there's another component in cannabis, a terpenoid called caryophyllene, that also is anti-addictive through a totally different mechanism than CBD. It's working on another receptor called the CB2 receptor that's involved in addiction. So, a preparation that had THC, CBD, and caryophyllene may be an ideal way of dealing with chronic pain and particularly people who are addicted to opioids.

Dr. Russo has the scientific background to make clear why he believes that CBD may be the power force needed to counteract the devastating effect of opioids in our country today. He believes that our efforts against opioids have produced lousy results so far because we've simply been using the wrong tools for the job . . . but CBD shows every promise of being the right tool. (As you can see, I also like Dr. Russo because I think he's an effective evangelist for the science that is leading this revolution.)

It's hard to sum up my deep respect for this man—or to make clear in just a few words why he is one of my personal heroes—but if there's one thing that drives both of us, I believe it's an unwillingness to be satisfied with the current state of things. Opioid-based treatments for pain have left the nation in a deep crisis that is literally destroying communities. Treatment for diseases like Alzheimer's and Parkinson's is "just okay" with some patients getting good results, but many are still left out in the cold. As our nation's Baby Boomer population ages,

Dr. Russo realizes that conditions related to aging are only going to get more prevalent. There will be more diagnoses, and more people are going to need all the help we can give them. Dr. Russo knows we can do better, and I strongly agree with that sentiment.

DR. AIDAN HAMPSON

Dr. Aidan Hampson is a program and scientific officer and special subject expert on cannabis and kratom in the Division of Therapeutic Development at the National Institute on Drug Abuse. He advises the NIDA leadership on cannabinoid and kratom science and coauthored a review on cannabis pharmacology with the NIDA Director, including the effect of cannabidiol across a range of preclinical seizure models. He has been studying cannabinoids seriously since 1994. Aidan was a Principal Scientist at Cortex Pharmaceuticals in Irvine, California, for eight years in early 2000, where he was responsible for the group conducting pharmacological characterization of new molecular entities and assay development. Aidan is a trained cannabinoid pharmacologist in the Pharmacology Department of UC San Francisco and also trained with Nobel Laureate Dr. Julius Axelrod (at the National Institute of Mental Health). He is also the first author of a groundbreaking US Patent titled "Cannabinoids as Neuroprotective Antioxidant."

Many of the scientists profiled here will be characterized as the "father" of something

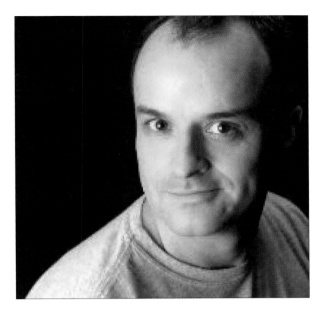

Dr. Aidan Hampson

related to CBD. In Dr. Hampson's case, he is truly the father of establishing that CBD can definitively function as an antioxidant. His patent—which was granted in 2003—makes clear the pharmaceutical compositions and compounds that can be used in neuroprotectants and cardioprotectants. Specifically, the patent is not for a particular strain of CBD or a related compound, but rather for "a method of treating diseases caused by oxidative stress, comprising administering a therapeutically effective amount of a cannabinoid that has substantially no binding to the NMDA receptor to a subject who has a disease caused by oxidative stress."

Dr. Hampson's stated goal with this innovation was to create a new class of antioxidant drugs that could act as neuroprotectants while also being useful in the treatment of associated diseases. The goal was also to design cannabinoid compounds that would be able to provide these treatments while being substantially free of any psychoactive effects, as well as safe and nontoxic at most dose levels.

In the application for the patent itself, Dr. Hampson includes the story of how he came to formulate this treatment:

> It has surprisingly been found that cannabidiol and other cannabinoids can function as neuroprotectants, even though they lack NMDA receptor antagonist activity. This discovery was made possible because of the inventor's recognition of a previously unanticipated antioxidant property of the cannabinoids in general (and cannabidiol in particular) that functions completely independently of antagonism at the NMDA, AMPA and kainate receptors. Hence the present invention includes methods of preventing or treating diseases caused by oxidative stress, such as neuronal hypoxia, by administering a prophylactic or therapeutically effective amount of a cannabinoid to a subject who has a disease caused by oxidative stress.

Dr. Hampson was saying that he was able to come up with this patentable treatment because he noticed a property of cannabinoids that nobody else had seen, namely, that they can function as an antioxidant by interacting with receptors that had not yet been studied. Later in the patent, Dr. Hampson mentions that he has high hopes for CBD in these treatments, noting it is "particularly advantageous to use because it avoids toxicity encountered with [other] cannabinoids (such as THC) at high doses." He states that CBD affects how you perceive THC in your body. Speaking to him most recently, we discussed a series of questions I wanted to ask all of our experts, with one of them being how he felt about the classification of CBD in general. Should it be classified as a supplement or a drug that is regulated by the FDA? "Dose makes the poison," he stated, and this quote was more true of CBD than anything else. Especially in regard to prescription drugs such as blood thinners. He said that without case studies it was difficult to state specific amounts, but that when taken at a therapeutic index, CBD seemed to enhance the results of certain drugs like Warfarin. We both agree that more research needs to be conducted and that the future of cannabinoids like CBD is looking hopeful. When asked where he saw the future of cannabis regulation or declassification, he mentioned that he felt we would see cannabis being descheduled, completely, at best.

After his influential patent, Hampson has continued to conduct groundbreaking work. In 2005, he undertook important work on the ability of CBD to counteract the effects of alcohol-induced brain damage. More recently, he has focused on CBD's impact on overall well-being. In fact, when I spoke to him more specifically about how he sees the various "delivery systems" available to the public, at this time, he mentioned that he felt like the "perfect" formulation or method did not exist yet, given the nature of how cannabinoids like CBD are processed in the body. The effective strategy in humans for optimal absorption is to combine your desired method like an oil tincture or softgel with a 7–10-gram serving of fat.

Yes, fat.

This is done to divert the normal processing procedure, conducted by the liver, and to briefly detour it to the lymphatic system by incorporating fat molecules. The fat molecules scoop up the cannabinoids and deliver them into the bloodstream before they enter the liver . . . which effectively prevents a majority of their destruction. There is an increase in absorption somewhere in the range of 300–400 percent when CBD is taken in this manner. Which goes right along with Dr. Russo's suggested Mediterranean diet, consisting of things like olive oils, fish, avocados, nuts, and cheeses.

In 2017, Dr. Hampson and other colleagues published an influential paper titled "Don't Worry, Be Happy: Endocannabinoids and Cannabis at the Intersection of Stress and Reward." This study examined the ways in which the endocannabinoid system can be stimulated to enhance a sense of satisfaction and modulate responses to stress. The authors noted that, historically, cannabis users would use the drug for its satisfying effects, but consequential neuroadaptations meant that the users gradually found themselves using more and more of the substance—in effect, forming a habit or addiction. But in this study, alternate stimulations of the endocannabinoid system—including by CBD—are studies as

alternatives that could help those who benefit from such stimulation find a route that is not habit-forming. Dr. Hampson is more specifically interested in the "bell-shaped curve" that happens in the body when one takes cannabinoids for an extended period of time. This curve is essentially the polar opposite of what traditional medicines do in the body, where they reach a plateau and then fall off or level out. This anomaly in the body is curious to most researchers in the field and something Dr. Hampson hopes to dive into further.

I feel that Dr. Aidan Hampson qualifies as a living legend in the CBD community. He could have stopped after his groundbreaking patent, and his reputation and legacy would have been secure. But that's not his style. He has continued to lead and innovate, and to ask the hard questions we still need answered. Because of this, he is very much an inspiration to me.

DR. ALEXANDROS MAKRIYANNIS

Another hero of mine is Dr. Alex Makriyannis, the chair of pharmaceutical biotechnology at Northeastern University in Boston, Massachusetts, and also the founder and director of the Center for Drug Discovery. Dr. Makriyannis earned a bachelor's degree in chemistry from the University of Cairo and a PhD in medicinal chemistry from the University of Kansas.

He is a highly successful medicinal chemist and is well recognized both nationally

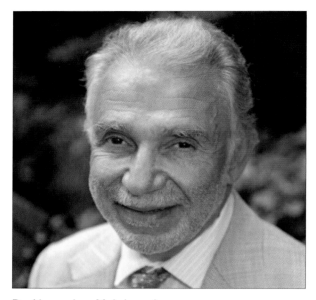

Dr. Alexandros Makriyannis

and internationally for his important contributions in endocannabinoid research. His forty-year contributions to laboratory design have catalyzed some of the key pharmacological endocannabinoid probes that are widely used today, while serving as leads for the development of new medications. Dr. Makriyannis has also made important contributions for understanding the molecular basis of cannabinoid activity and has been a creative pioneer in the field of chemical biology, where his work has been recognized for its high level of originality. Some of his compounds are in advanced preclinical trials for the treatment of metabolic disorders and liver function, neuropathic pain, addiction, and neurodegenerative diseases.

It's hard to identify which of Dr. Makriyannis's accomplishments are the most meaningful—and this is not least because they are still coming at a remarkable pace!

In 2016, for example, I was cheered when he published important findings in the journal *Cell* that seemed to open the door to new understandings of the way cannabinoids have the potential to impact conditions like pain and obesity. What Dr. Makriyannis had done was to identify the three-dimensional structure of CB1 for the first time. The project, which took years of work and collaboration, is now allowing medicines and treatments acting on CB1 to be better targeted. Put more specifically, the 3D model will allow drugs to be "stickier" and "more adhesive" when they interact with CB1. They will fit with it more perfectly and stick to it for a greater duration. Previous drugs that might have produced a moderate interaction with CB1—think of it as like a "glancing blow"—will now be able to aim for something more like a "direct hit." For example, a drug that targets CB1 and currently eliminates chemotherapy pain moderately and temporarily could be adjusted to act more powerfully and for a longer period of time.

Dr. Makriyannis is also allowing us to better understand CBD and THC with an eye to increasing product safety. Because CBD and THC so often exist in a regulatory and legal "gray zone" in many communities, finding ways to keep products safe is of vital importance. Many instances of "bad press" suffered by CBD and THC in recent years have arisen from consumers using illegal and unsafe synthetic cannabinoids, like Spice and K-2. These synthetics are ripe for abuse, have many side effects, and have even proven fatal in some cases.

"But isn't that all the same stuff?" an ill-informed member of the public might ask. "Isn't that all just cannabinoids, whether they're synthetic or otherwise?"

Dr. Makriyannis's research allows us to say, "No," and to do so definitively.

Through his research and understanding of the CB1 binding and activation mechanism, we are learning precisely why natural CBD and THC are safe, and why synthetics are not.

Dr. Makriyannis and his team used X-ray crystallography to analyze the binding process of molecules interacting with CB1. (X-ray crystallography turns individual molecules into crystals, right when they're in the middle of doing something important—like binding to CB1. Because crystallization creates data that researchers can use to reconstruct a picture of what a molecule is doing at a certain point in time, it allows them to "see" molecules and their functions in ways a typical microscope could not.) This new research showed that CB1 receptors shrank when interacting with certain molecules, which meant that they could be encouraged to react in ways that had never before been envisioned. Not only does it mean that synthetic cannabinoids are likely interacting with CB1 cells in a *totally different way* from regular cannabis, but that more precise targeting of CB1 interactions for medicinal purposes is definitely possible.

Today, Dr. Makriyannis is leading the fight for more research in a number of ways. He is the head of the Center for Drug Discovery, an organization with the mission of developing new drugs from the cannabinoid system. This center brings together industry-leading researchers and pharmacologists to develop new medications and also continue to study how cannabis works in relation to THC and CBD. He is especially interested in trichomes, which he calls the "engine" of cannabinoids: bioactive molecules that can work in many different conditions. Makriyannis believes that by understanding the basic building blocks of cannabinoids—and cannabinoid biosynthesis—additional useful discoveries can be made. He is also working to isolate and understand the root differences of CBD and THC, which, as he is always quick to point out, are separated by a single oxygen molecule. In addition to this new research, he has continued studying the placement of CB1 and CB2 receptors throughout the body. Since 2002, he has been interested in how CB1 and CB2 could be manipulated to play a role in helping people overcome addiction and substance abuse. He has stated that with the latest advancements, the technology now exists to "turn off" CB1 receptors. A treatment that did this would, for example, be able to block the intoxicating effects of cannabis use for someone who was addicted to it.

Though he is now eighty years old, Dr. Makriyannis is still going strong. His career and accomplishments have been recognized throughout the globe, and he has been presented with numerous awards in his field. In addition to personal accolades, he has been instrumental to many important boards and is on the editorial board of no fewer than five journals in his field. He remains one of my heroes in the field, and I'm so excited to see what he will do next.

DR. RAPHAEL MECHOULAM

A man who would certainly be a strong candidate for "most important CBD researcher ever," Dr. Raphael Mechoulam was one of the first international research scientists to challenge the suppression of hemp and the endocannabinoid system. At the time, his work was labeled radical and unsavory, when in reality he was brilliantly ahead of his time. His

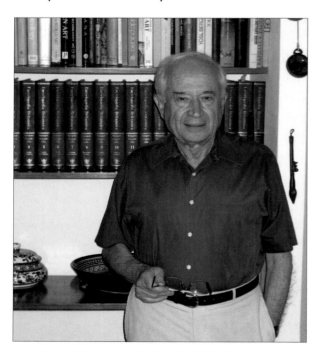

Warrior and Innovator Dr. Raphael Mechoulam.

research over a decade ago led to a medicinal revolution in hemp cannabinoids.

Dr. Mechoulam was born in Sofia, Bulgaria, in 1930, and his personal story combating adversity and challenge is—I believe—key to understanding how and why he has become such an effective advocate for CBD. He was born to a Jewish family in the height of the anti-Semitism that was rampant in the run-up to World War II. At various times, his family had to move because of anti-Jewish prejudice, and his father narrowly survived being sent to a concentration camp. Some would say his fate after the war was also difficult because of Bulgaria's subsequent takeover by the Soviets.

Nonetheless, Dr. Mechoulam stayed motivated and focused. He earned a degree in biochemistry from the Hebrew University of Jerusalem, and then a doctorate at the Weizmann Institute of Science in Rehovot, Israel (a leading university that only offers graduate degrees in the sciences). From there, his groundbreaking research into the effects of cannabinoids has won him multiple honorary doctorates, as well as many of the major prizes and awards in the sciences. He deserves the accolades, as his work is simply remarkable.

In 1963, while working at the Hebrew University, he became the first person to isolate THC. Later quoted at his office in the Department of Medicinal Chemistry and Natural Products at the Hadassah-Hebrew University medical school, he explains that scientists as far back as the 1800s realized the beneficial effects of hemp, but political problems stifled any serious study. "I believe that cannabinoids represent a medicinal treasure trove which waits to be discovered." In 1964, he won the Somach Sachs Prize for "best research by a scientist below age thirty-five" at the Weizmann Institute. By the 1990s, Raphael was a prominent figure in the hemp cannabinoid world, achieving a dedication in the monthly issue of "Pharmacology, Biochemistry and Behavior" for achievements in the cannabinoid field, as well as being elected Member of the Israeli Academy of Sciences. The International Cannabinoid Research Society has recognized him for his efforts in the field, and, in 1999, they dedicated an annual award to be named "The R. Mechoulam." Later, in 2007, they gave him the lifetime achievement award in cannabinoid research. His passion for hemp has led to the development of many control studies and has become the blueprint for many clinical trials still used today.

Many call Dr. Mechoulam the Father (or Grandfather) of cannabidiol research. When he began his work, powerful drugs like opium and cocaine had already had their chemistry isolated—with their underpinning mechanisms relatively well understood—while cannabis was still basically a mystery. People who used it could tell you how it made them feel, but the active compounds had not been isolated. Yet just as tremendously valuable medicines and painkillers had been derived through the understanding of other drugs, Dr. Mechoulam understood that there could be a tremendous

benefit to grasping the underlying features of cannabis. (In interviews, Dr. Mechoulam has said that he was intrigued by a story he'd once heard about a poet in the Middle East in the 1400s whose son suffered from seizures. The story went that the poet eventually gave his son hashish, and the seizures stopped. However, the son had to continue using the substance to stay seizure-free. It's not known if this story is true, but it's interesting that this story may have been the catalyst to so many important scientific discoveries to come.)

To plumb the depths of cannabis, he knew the necessity to start at the beginning . . . which is exactly what he did. Yet the discoveries and innovations came quickly—a testament, I believe, to his foresight and intelligence. Not long after identifying the structure of cannabidiol, he had isolated THC for the first time. He also helped to establish and isolate many of the other compounds found in cannabis, including reisolating CBD. (CBD had first been isolated back in 1940 by Alexander Todd and Roger Adams.)

However, his work did not stop when these compounds were isolated. He continued to devote himself to unraveling the scientific mysteries behind the cannabis plant. For example, in the '60s and '70s, the way THC "worked" was not completely understood. Researchers knew it was the thing producing the most noticeable effect in marijuana users, but how? At the time, many thought THC was metabolized by a cell membrane. Yet Dr. Mechoulam and his team were able to show that, in actuality, the THC was acting through a specific mechanism and found the compounds that were interacting with cannabinoid receptors.

His recent work has involved looking into the phenolic acids that are produced by cannabis and that contain CBD or THC. Previous investigations of these acids have been difficult because they are active and break down. However, Dr. Mechoulam is using chemical modifications to make them stable and in doing so is searching for new uses and applications for them. In speaking with him, I discovered research I had not come across previously, and I felt it was important to share the discussion we had and to include the studies he shared with me, so that you could look them up for yourself, next time you are in a debate with someone who doesn't think cannabis is medicine.

Our conversation is as follows:

Q: What cannabinoids do you think have the most profound effect on mankind?
A: Presumably anandamide and 2-AG (endogenous cannabinoids), which are involved in a large number of physiological processes and diseases. For example:

D. Panikashvili, C. Simeonidou, S. Ben-Shabat, L. Hanus, A. Breuer, R. Mechoulam and E. Shohami. An endogenous cannabinoid (2-AG) is neuroprotective after brain injury. Nature 413, 527-531 (2001).
Q: What research currently being conducted excites you the most?

A: My own (of course; what do you expect?). There are about 100 anandamide–like compounds in the body that seem to be involved in a huge number of effects.

For example:

G. Milman, Y. Maor, S. Abu-Lafi, M. Horowitz, R. Gallily, S. Batkai, F-M. Mo, L. Offertaler, P. Pacher, G. Kunos, R. Mechoulam. N-Arachidonoyl L-serine, a novel endocannabinoid-like brain constituent with vasodilatory properties. Proc Natl Acad Sci US A, 103, 2428-2433 (2006).

R. Smoum, A. Bar, B. Tan, G. Milman, M. Attar-Namdar, O. Ofek, J.M. Stuart, A. Bajayo, Y. Tam, V. Kram, D. O'Dell, M. J. Walker, H. B. Bradshaw, I. Bab, R. Mechoulam. Oleoyl serine, an endogenous regulator of skeletal mass. Proc Natl Acad Sci US A. 107, 17710-5 (2010).

M. Feldman, R. Smoum, R. Mechoulam, D. Steinberg. Antimicrobial potential of endocannabinoid and endocannabinoid-like compounds against methicillin-resistant Staphylococcus aureus. Sci Rep. 8, 17696 (2018).

S. Baraghithy, S. R. Smoum, R. A. Drori, A. R. Hadar, R. A. Gammal, A. S. Hirsch, M. Attar-Namdar, A. Nemirovski, Y. Gabet, Y. Langer, Y. Pollak, C. P. Schaaf, M. E. Rech, V. Gross-Tsur, I. Bab, R. Mechoulam, J. Tam. Magel2 Modulates Bone Remodeling and Mass in Prader-Willi Syndrome by Affecting Oleoyl Serine Levels and Activity. J Bone Miner Res. 34, 93-105 (2019).

G. Donvito, F. Piscitelli, P. Muldoon, A. Jackson, R. Vitale, E. D'Aniello, C. Giordano, B. Ignatowska-Jankowska, M. Mustafa,

F. Guida, G.P etrie, L. Parker, R. Smoum, L. J. Sim-Selley, S. Maione, A. H. Lichtman, M. I. Damaj, V. Di Marzo, R. Mechoulam. N-Oleoyl glycine reduces nicotine reward and withdrawal in mice. Neuropharmacol. 148, 320-331 (2019).

Some of this research is truly cutting-edge, and I encourage you to check it out for yourself. Dr Mechoulam mentioned that he felt that for most people to gain significant relief using a CBD supplement, dosing should range somewhere between 250–800mg daily, which is conducive to some of the other opinions we have heard in this book. We are very excited to be connected with him and see what's next on the horizon for cannabinoids as a whole.

TRACY RYAN

Tracy is the CEO and lead consultant for CannaKids, a California-based cooperative with a focus on supplying medical cannabis oil to adults and children looking for holistic relief in serious health conditions, like cancer and epilepsy. She has been featured in *National Geographic*, CNN, *Fox Business*, *Entertainment Tonight*, and in several international publications for her contributions to the pediatric community. Inspired by the desire for a more natural approach to her infant daughter's cancer diagnosis in 2013 and armed with a true passion for clinical research, she has partnered with—and is on the advisory board of CURE, a leading disruptive drug delivery technology company with a focus on pharmaceutical

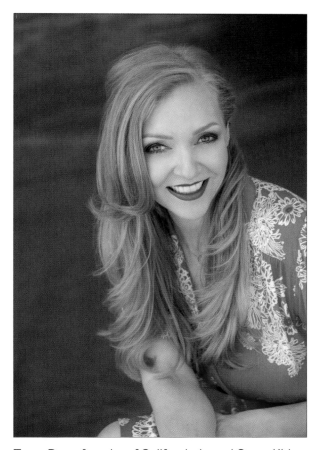

Tracy Ryan, founder of California-based CannaKids.

cannabinoid molecule development; and the Technion Institute in Israel, who is leading the way for cannabis research in cancer. Her dedication and research in Israel has paved the way for the beginning phases of in-hospital clinical trials that are being conducted with pediatric cancer patients in California. Tracy can be found speaking at medical practices all over the world about the health benefits and her research with hemp cannabinoids.

Tracy is important to the CBD movement, as her story is so relatable. Even in 2019, many Americans view cannabis and products derived from it as "the other," as something

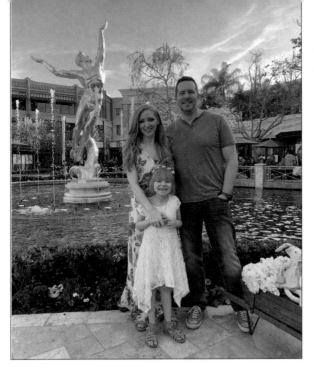

Tracy Ryan and family pose in celebration of Sophie's incredible journey and success using cannabinoids as medicine.

that is transgressive and potentially unsafe—outside of the sphere of "healthy and normal" interests.

Here to shatter that stereotype is Tracy Ryan.

It's one thing for a scientist in a white lab coat to give a presentation about the chemical properties of cannabis and the pharmaceutical possibilities to be derived therefrom. While scientists speak with authority, they are not always relatable. Unless we also work in the sciences, they may seem possessed of a way of viewing the world that is lost to us. But it is quite another thing when someone like Tracy Ryan tells her story.

Her story starts in the mid-2010s, when her daughter, Sophie, was diagnosed with a brain tumor. Tracy Ryan set out to educate herself on the condition, and to figure out what to do next. As any parent would be, she was devastated by the diagnosis but determined to do everything within her power to help her daughter.

Physicians initially said that Sophie's only hope lay in a 13-month regimen of chemotherapy. Sophie's tumor was such that her body would never be rid of it, they said, though they believed it would be possible to slow or stop its growth.

As so many do in the twenty-first century, Tracy used social media to spread the word about what her daughter was facing. She wanted to keep friends and relatives informed, she wanted support, but she also wanted to send out feelers for anything that might be useful for the hard road ahead. Tracy started the Facebook page "Prayers for Sophie," and a friend on the social network put her in touch with the talk show host Ricki Lake and filmmaker Abby Epstein. The pair was making a documentary about the positive health impacts of cannabis and the healing potentials that lay within it.

With help from Lake and Epstein, Tracy set about educating herself on the health benefits that cannabinoids might hold for her daughter.

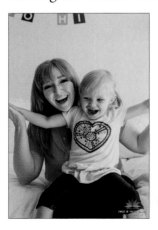
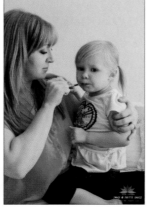

Despite being in an almost constant battle for her life, Sophie's immune system is stronger than that of the average healthy adult, thanks to hemp cannabinoids.

Shortly thereafter, Sophie began a regimen of THC and CBD concentrate in addition to her chemotherapy . . . and Tracy found that the results were phenomenal.

Sophie did not face many of the side effects usually caused by chemotherapy; she did not lose weight and maintained a healthy appetite. The only side effect from the THC–CBD concentrate seemed to be moderate sleepiness, and this side effect receded as Sophie grew acclimated to it.

After the thirteen months of powerful anti-cancer drugs, Sophie's doctors were happy to report that her brain tumor had done more than stop growing—it had shrunk by about 90 percent. In addition, a cyst that had also formed was about 90 percent reduced.

But that wasn't all. Sophie's physicians had told her that even with successful treatment, because of the positions of the tumor and the cyst, she would probably lose all sight in her left eye and have reduced vision in her right. However, her vision was not impacted at all.

And most remarkably, months after her last chemotherapy treatment, Sophie's doctors found that her tumor had disappeared entirely. According to Tracy, Sophie's physicians believe that this disappearance of the tumor—and the total preservation of her eyesight—may be explained by her continued use of THC and CBD.

Many people might have been forgiven for stopping their involvement with cannabinoids at this point. Sophie had been cured of her tumor, and she had identified a course of THC –CBD that appeared ready to serve her well going forward. Tracy was doubtless exhausted by the trauma of her daughter's health episode. Many mothers would simply have thanked their stars that their daughter had been cured and beat a path back to trying to have a "normal life."

But not Tracy Ryan.

When her daughter experienced a positive health outcome, it only motivated Tracy to become *more* involved in opening the public's eyes to the tremendous possibilities awaiting in THC and CBD.

So she started her company, CannaKids, to focus on supplying medical cannabis oil to both adults and children, though specializing in patients with pediatric cancer. This organization is now one of the global leaders in cannabis information. She has also aggressively advocated partnerships between CannaKids and researchers and tech companies who are developing new ways of delivering THC and CBD. I don't think it is overstating things to say that Tracy has become a "cannabis disruptor" in more than one area.

Tracy is doing so much that it is hard to keep up with all of her accomplishments and projects. In 2019, she worked on expanding her CannaKids brand to Canada and Australia, and Europe may be next (while she also investigates the Asian market). In addition, she has taken a role in advocating to train nurses on working with patients who use CBD or THC therapies.

Tracy says that her stretch goal would be

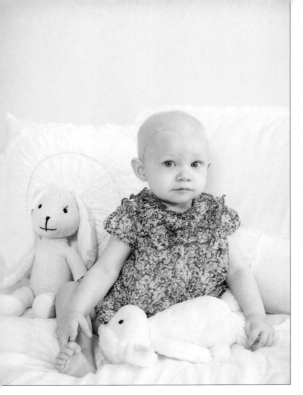

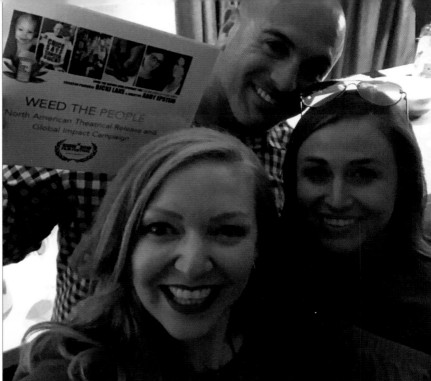

Tracy knew cannabis was helping Sophie and became determined to see other children successfully beating cancer

Ryan Lewis with Tracy Ryan and Amanda Rice at the private viewing party for *Weed the People*.

to open cannabinoid-based "wellness clinics" within the next few years throughout all major cities. These would be centers for treatment and education, and places where parents could walk in and learn about the benefits of CBD and THC for their families.

While many organizations are now working to connect parents seeking more information with the top research on THC and CBD, Tracy has the added benefit of having been there herself. She knows what it is like to be a mother whose child may be dying. She has dealt with doctors and nurses who have varying degrees of receptiveness to CBD and THC and has seen how the attitudes of medical professionals can change over time. And she also knows the good news. For her, of course, it's personal. She is able to share Sophie's story with parents who have questions . . . and they have a lot of questions.

I asked Tracy some questions I wanted to highlight for the book, such as which research excites her the most, and did she take any cannabinoid products herself? Which cannabinoids did she think had the most profound effect on mankind? She was eager to respond and help people to understand the truly magical aspects of cannabinoids.

"We all know about THC and CBD, both of which are extremely therapeutic in both our observational studies and our clinical research. But molecules like CBDa, THCa, CBG, and CBN are getting a lot of attention. We have been using CBDa for our cancer patients, THCa has been vastly used by our Autism, ADD & ADHD community, CBG also for cancer patients, and CBN is amazing for sleep from what we have observed. Our research, not to sound biased, is probably the most exciting

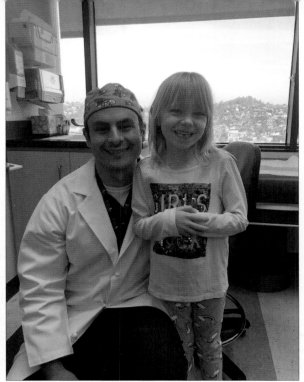

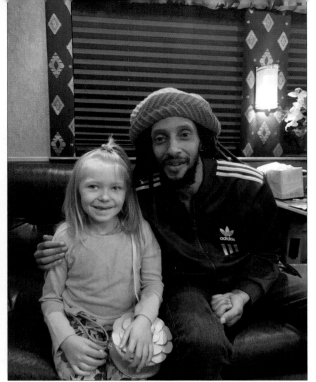

Sophie makes friends at UCLA with her infectious energy while being treated by some of the best doctors in the world.

Sophie visits with cannabis supporter Ziggy Marley at the *Weed the People* premiere.

to me. We currently have nineteen patients enrolled in groundbreaking research led by world-renowned immunologist Dr. Anahid Jewett. We just filed our provisional patent showing that cannabis is killing cancer stem cells, and even chemo and radiation can't do that. This will be very big news in the coming year as we begin to announce it more widely in the media. We have also filed a patent showing that cannabis is reactivating the Natural Killer Cell System, which is the driver of our innate immune system. In Dr. Jewett's thirty-year career, she has discovered that it's the failure of this system that leads us to get cancer in the first place. We now have a clear-cut path to human trials that we intend to stay on until we can get therapeutics to the market and into the hands of doctors. I am hopeful that we will be able to prove that this plant should be consumed every

day of your life as a preventative to cancer, and also a very powerful tool in the tool belts of cancer patients who are currently battling this disease. For folks who are looking to take a daily, I recommend everyone take at least 50mg. per day, in upward of 150 if illness is a concern. For those in chronic pain, dosage recommendations can get tricky. It depends on the degree of pain. I can take a very large dose and it will affect me one way, and a dose the 16th of the size will affect my husband in the exact same way even though he's much bigger than I. We all metabolize drugs differently. A range could be 40–70mg., 3 times a day. I take CBD and THC every single day of my life, and I have a lot of pain from all of my years of sports and dance. I used to have arthritis until it disappeared after I consumed high doses of cannabis daily. Due to there being research showing that this is possible, this is what I attribute my recovery and current well-being to, since I don't take anything else at all. Reversing arthritis isn't something that just happens, either. I also use it to help me sleep, to shut down the noise in my head, for pain from injuries, and to block my nightmares and bad memories after having gone through six years of pediatric cancer with my little girl. It's amazing how one plant can help me in so many different ways, and keep me off of pharmaceutical drugs that are addictive and can be harmful."

Something I discussed with doctors in the field, that I felt Tracy would have an educated opinion on, is how CBD should be classified. Should it be regulated as a drug or as a plant-based supplement?

Tracy said, "Currently it should definitely

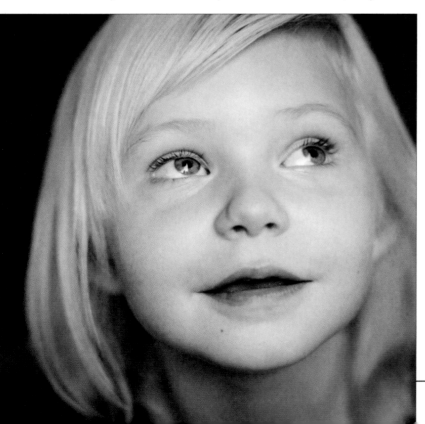

be regulated as a plant-based supplement. This is truly a medicine though, at certain dosages, so holding clinical trials in order to get regulated and scientific will help develop proven meds that can be overseen by the FDA, so insurance can cover the high costs. But it should definitely *not* be taken out of the people's hands for personal use."

Until her dream of calculated and accessible wellness clinics becomes a reality, Tracy is passionate about reaching out to doctors and nurses to educate them about the benefits of cannabinoids. As she shares virtually, whenever she is interviewed, Tracy is still astounded to regularly meet physicians in top hospitals who are resistant to cannabinoid treatments in children, or who have a complete lack of knowledge about them. She is passionate about trying to change minds and has made her website SavingSophie.org into a network of research designed to change minds. Visitors can learn about the hard science behind CBD and THC, and her personal story—yes—but they'll also find information about cancer charities, different types of cancers, nutrition and cancer, and resources on getting involved in clinical trials.

Speaking candidly, Tracy says, "My daughter has been using CBD and THC for over six years for her brain tumor, Epilepsy and for immune system

Beautiful Sophie continues to fight every day, giving hope to other children like her, all because of her incredible family and their belief in the healing power of hemp cannabinoids.

stimulation. She's been an incredible case study on how beneficial this plant can be, and every doctor that has treated her has seen the benefits first-hand. She drives everything I have ever done in regard to cannabis. She inspired us to create CannaKids and SavingSophie. org. She's my cohost on our new iTunes podcast called Saving Sophie, and our research all started because of her. I am on a mission to work with Dr. Jewett and her team of scientists, to not only irradiate Soph's tumor, but also help aid other patients like her."

I feel like if someone asked, "Is Tracy Ryan changing the world through massive projects or is she doing it one person at a time?" the only honest answer would be "Yes." Tracy is doing both. At the same time.

Here's hoping she never stops.

RICK SIMPSON

Thanks to the highly successful documentary *Run From the Cure*, Rick Simpson became a household name in the cannabinoid world almost overnight. While studies have long been reported for the antitumor-like effects of hemp cannabinoids, it really wasn't mainstream conversation until his documentary began highlighting the magic of CBD in conjunction with THC. Simpson had been interested in hemp cannabinoids since his cousin's bout with cancer in 1969, as he witnessed the results from chemotherapy. The Rick Simpson oil has cured, given relief to, and sent to remission a slew of cancerous processes

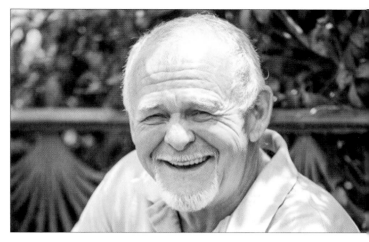

Rick Simpson

with its developmental roots originating in a Canadian hospital where he worked.

One of the most inspiring things about Simpson is his vision—and history shows that every movement needs visionaries. They can show us what a future might look like, if only we have the resolve and energy to take the steps needed to get there.

He believes in a world in which everyone has easy access to the healing properties of THC and CBD. He feels passionately that there should be no barriers against consumers growing their own cannabis and/or help, and with the proper knowledge creating their own CBD or THC products for personal use. I get the feeling that Simpson views it the way many people think about grocery stores. Groceries make it easy to buy your own fruits and vegetables with very little effort, but nobody would dream of a world where government regulations said we *forbid* you from growing your own kale and green beans, or having a lemon tree in your yard. That would be ridiculous. Because cannabis has been proven to be so safe and so salutary, Simpson believes the government should trust us with it the same way they trust us with a green bean or a lemon.

Simpson uses the word *medicine* to refer to cannabis. That's also key to understanding his perspective and how he believes cannabinoids can change the world. He believes that hemp oil can be produced safely by consumers and that, given time, growing your own hemp and extracting useful THC or CBD from it can become as commonplace as someone harvesting and preparing food they've grown in a home garden.

In *Run From the Cure*, Simpson profiled Americans who have suffered from everything—chronic back pain to panic attacks to pain related to major surgeries. Skin allergies and skin cancers also figure prominently. Each one of them have had positive results from homemade hemp oil.

Some of the testimonials Simpson uses are clearly cases that run to the extreme and that require further study—such as testimonials from people who had been given only weeks to live by a physician but experienced essentially miraculous cures after using hemp oil with CBD and THC. (Clearly, someone with a dire diagnosis cannot expect CBD or THC to work in every case, and Rick takes care not to represent these instances as guaranteed to work for everyone. It's clear that they are often few and far between. But they do exist and they *are* real, and I think it's vital that Simpson give them a voice and a platform.)

Simpson also does an excellent job of explaining for everyday Americans the wide range of possibilities for hemp oil, and all the areas of the body that CBD can potentially help with. (My favorite line from *Run From the Cure* might be when he says: "I would like someone to tell me what it *can't* heal!")

Simpson also has made a commitment not to profit personally from CBD oil. This is not a decision he necessarily has to make, but he is passionate about the idea that everyone should understand that he is not "in it for the money." His motivations—his *only* motivations—are to see CBD help as many people as it possibly can, and to smash the negative stereotypes that still exist.

For Simpson, the journey to CBD is as personal as it could be. The way he became the man he is today helps me to understand why he has such a need for his intentions to appear earnest and genuine.

In 1972, Rick Simpson's brother died from cancer. Just three years after his brother's death, Rick was listening to the radio and heard a broadcast about a researcher who claimed that THC could kill cancer. However, he never heard any follow-up broadcasts about this cancer cure and assumed that the claims had subsequently been proved untrue. In 1997, Simpson himself suffered a serious head injury with aftereffects related to concussions. At the time, his physicians put him on the best medicines available. However, he was still unsatisfied. The aftereffects of his injury were not totally controlled, and he suffered from unpleasant side effects brought on by the medication. Then, in 1997, he viewed a television program that profiled people who'd had good luck improving their health, and minimizing the impacts of health conditions, by using cannabis. Thinking that he had nothing to lose, Rick purchased some cannabis and began experimenting with personal use. He found that it improved his postinjury symptoms better than any of the pills he'd been given, and with no side effects.

The seeds of hemp evangelism began to grow inside Simpson. He went back to his physicians and shared the positive impact that cannabis had on his symptoms. But when he asked them if they could prescribe him cannabis and incorporate it into his postinjury treatment, they refused. Instead, they cautioned him that it was "understudied," and more than one physician cautioned that it could be bad for his lungs in the same way when inhaling cigarette smoke.

Determined not to give up, Simpson did some research on the ways cannabis could be deployed. Then he went back to his physicians and posed a question to them. If cannabis could be taken by ingesting it in the form of hemp oil, then wouldn't that eliminate the purported risk to his lungs?

His family doctor was somewhat won over, agreeing that hemp ingested in this format would indeed eliminate any risk to his lungs. However, the doctor still refused to help Rick acquire cannabis legally—still insisting that the effects were just too understudied.

This was when Simpson decided to take matters into his own hands. He began acquiring hemp on his own and making his own hemp oil, using it to treat himself.

Meanwhile, years went by, and in 2001 he was informed by his physicians that they knew of nothing further in established medical science that could be done to treat his head injury. He was—as they say—"now on his own." But Simpson continued making and taking his own hemp oil and continued to have positive results treating his pain. Simpson discontinued using the pills prescribed by his physician and only took the hemp oil. His condition continued to improve. He felt better, and people in his personal life told him he seemed like he was much improved. Was the hemp oil curing his condition? Was he "doing better" because he was now free from the side effects of the prescription medication? Or was it some combination of the two? Whatever the case, Rick liked what he was experiencing.

Then, a year later, Simpson noticed something new happening on his body—something that happens to millions of people, especially as they age—a thing that was serious, but not necessarily life-threatening. He had developed some spots on his face and body where a lifetime of exposure to the sun had accumulated. He knew that these were more than just freckles. They were the kind of spots that could be cancerous or precancerous, and that he should have a physician treat.

So, dutifully, Simpson went back to his doctor, who confirmed the spots required treatment. The doctor said that the most serious spot needed to be cut out right away, so he had a minor operation to remove it. However, he was curious about what would (or could) be done about the two other areas on his skin that his doctor had said would soon also require treatment. Drawing upon his own independent research about the healing effects of cannabis, he began applying a highly concentrated form of hemp oil to his other spots each day. To Simpson's delight—but perhaps not to his surprise—the other spots gradually disappeared completely.

It's important for me to say here that Rick Simpson did the right thing when he found these spots on his skin. He went to his doctor. When the doctor said one of the spots needed an operation immediately, he had the operation performed. Only then did Simpson use hemp oil on his other spots, which his doctor had told him did not yet constitute a medical emergency. (I want to be clear throughout this book that *nobody* should ever put off a surgery recommended by a physician to fix a life-threatening condition. However, seeing what cannabinoids can do for things that are not immediate medical emergencies—as more and more people are seeing each day—can sometimes result in experiences very close to Simpson's.)

This experience with the spots on his face led him to believe that just about everybody would be pleased to hear about his positive experience with hemp oil, and that it would be a good step in helping to convince members of the medical community of the beneficial effects of cannabis. Yet he still met with resistance. Simpson then tried to escalate things by investigating what it would take to go "over the head" of his doctor and get the Canadian government to allow him to legally possess cannabis and make hemp oil. Ironically, in addition to facing an approval process that would take nearly two years—and that by no means ensured he would be granted permission—the first step he would need would be a letter from his doctor endorsing the idea.

Consequently, Simpson resolved to become something of an outlaw. And when the authorities began cracking down on what he was doing, he decided to become a very public one.

Simpson grew cannabis on his own property and used it to make hemp oil. He used the hemp oil to treat himself and also gave some to his friends and neighbors. Many of the friends and neighbors also reported remarkable health improvements and relief from serious medical conditions as a consequence of its use. Eventually, law enforcement got wind of what he was doing and decided he could not be permitted to so openly defy the laws against cannabis. Although they did not arrest or fine him, the Royal Canadian Mounted Police conducted a raid on his property and removed all of his cannabis plants. That was when he decided to go public.

Believing that most people would be sympathetic to his story and what he was trying to do for his community, Simpson contacted media outlets across Canada and invited them to tell his story. Several took him up on it. He was honest, making sure to not exaggerate details or conceal others. He told the truth about what he had done and what the police had done. He also told the truth about the positive impacts that his homemade hemp oil was having on himself and others. His friends and neighbors also provided positive testimonials for the news cameras on the ways Simpson's hemp oil had helped them and their relatives. There were now dozens of people in the local community using the oil.

Rick Simpson thought that surely this sort of attention could only bolster interest in his hemp oil and help him to be taken seriously. He didn't know it at the time, but he was about to find out just how deep the prejudices against hemp and hemp oil ran.

Simpson and the community of supporters that soon assembled around him used his branch of the Royal Canadian Legion—a veteran's organization—as a kind of headquarters for their movement. He spoke about the benefits of hemp oil at the legion, and most of the members from his local post supported him. These members wrote petitions to the government and to the national headquarters of the Legion urging them to come to Simpson's local branch and see his cures firsthand. He and his supporters believed that if they could gradually win over Legion members from across Canada, it could be a first step to winning over other national organizations. Instead, the opposite happened. When the Legion received word of what he was doing, they shut down his local branch!

Unwilling to look at the evidence of his cures, the national organization chose to view what was happening through an entirely different lens—one that is all too familiar to early proponents of cannabis, THC, and CBD as medicine. They said they believed that Simpson was simply promoting "illegal drugs" and that this stood to damage the reputation of the Legion.

This was a major setback for Simpson, but he was determined to push forward. He began making his own video guides to the manufacturing of hemp oil. As we all know, technology changes everything. Simpson knew that this was true regarding the technology that allowed him to create hemp oil, but also true for the dissemination of information. He so firmly believed that if he could get the word out to other communities—across Canada and the world—then other people would come to find that they too could experience its positive effects. The government might be able to shut down one isolated group of evangelists for hemp oil operating out of a lone veteran's hall, but what if he could "plant the seeds" for hemp oil everywhere? By making video guides with instructions and testimonials, Rick started getting the word out about the effects of CBD oil.

This culminated in the production of his documentary film *Run From the Cure*, which became a viral way of telling his personal story and the story of hemp oil. In this intensely personal film, Simpson not only explores the healing effects of hemp oil, but also considers the growing rates of cancer around the world and the environmental factors that may be causing them. He challenges the viewers of his documentary to think for themselves and to take back agency when it comes to cannabis, while making some bold claims in his documentary and elsewhere. For example, he once told *High Times* magazine that his oil has an astounding 70 percent success rate for curing all types of cancer. This claim has not been studied or independently verified. Yet if even a fraction of his claims are true—and I have a feeling that they certainly are—then it's another strong case that more research needs to be done and that cannabinoids have the potential to help millions and millions of people.

His efforts to legitimize and distribute his CBD oil legally failed, but by getting the word out—simply telling his own story—he has made an immeasurable impact on cannabis culture, on science, and on society at large. Simpson's story makes me think of that line from *Star Wars* where Obi-Wan Kenobi is dueling with Darth Vader, and he says: "You can't win, Vader. If you strike me down, I shall become more powerful than you can possibly imagine."

Well, that happened.

Though the Royal Canadian Mounted Police struck down Simpson's ability to grow his hemp plants, his story made an impact so powerful, it is still being felt today!

Few advocates for cannabinoids can say that a cannabis-related product has actually been named after them. But he can. In the parlance of many in the marketplace, concentrated cannabis oil is now simply known as "Rick Simpson Oil." It is a loving tribute to his tireless work and advocacy, and something that I believe will outlive him for some time to come.

In closing, I will say that the thing I might like most about Rick Simpson is his humility. In his book, *Rick Simpson Oil: Nature's Answer for Cancer*, he describes his role in the grand scheme of things:

> . . . it does appear that I am the first to supply this medication to vast numbers of patients to treat their cancers and other conditions in a more effective and sensible way. In addition, I continued to report my findings openly to the general public after the government and all they control turned their backs on this issue. Since this plan has been used in medicine for thousands of years, I really do not think that anyone can make the claim that they alone discovered its true medical values. The only thing that I can really claim is that I discovered the proper way to produce and use this substance and I developed and published a protocol to make it more simple for patients to enjoy its use. As often as I could, I provided the medicine free of charge and I openly reported my findings to anyone who would listen, expecting that sooner or later someone would do something about it.

A class act all the way, and modest almost to a fault—that's how I think of Rick Simpson. He is a man whose contribution to the cause will be felt for generations. And I hope Rick knows that the world is starting to listen very closely to what he has been saying all along.

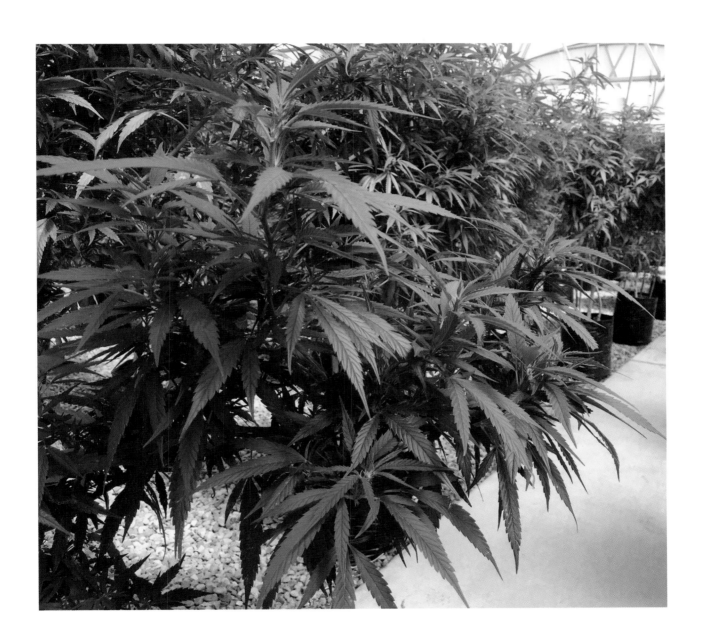

CHAPTER FOUR
GETTING STARTED WITH CBD: HOW TO USE IT AND WHAT TO LOOK FOR

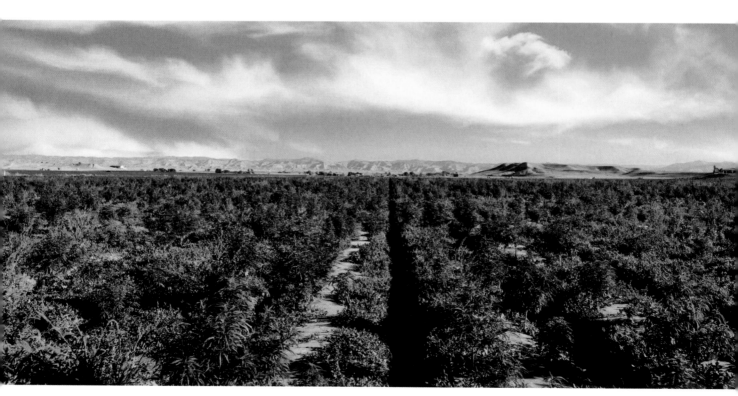

It may be that you are reading this book in hopes that I will get around to the specifics of your using CBD (and are annoyed that it had taken me this long!). Or it may be that you have read thus far as a skeptic, but I am beginning to convince you.

Whatever your situation, what I intend to lay out in this chapter are the facts about the choices now available for consumers when it comes to CBD. What is available now, what has been available, and what I expect we will see in the future.

Because CBD is new, the profession of a "CBD guide" is also relatively new. However, as each day passes there are more and more of us—and each day we know a little bit more than we did the day before. I hope you will also understand that everyone's experience with CBD is personal and unique. I will be able to tell you what works for most people, what only a few people enjoy, and so forth—but I will not be able to tell you precisely what your journey with CBD will be like. (Beware anyone who says that they can!)

But what I *can* promise you is that in this chapter I will try to be as useful as I possibly can. That I will speak plainly and in a straightforward way. And that I will try to answer the practical questions that people new to CBD actually want to know. (This isn't a place to try and show off my CBD knowledge, and I'll keep that in mind.)

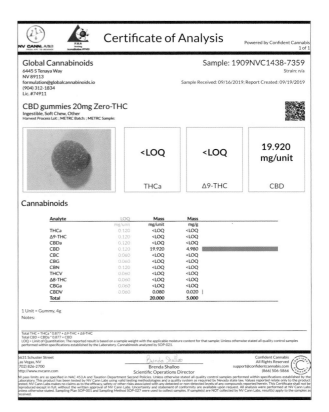

Certificate of Analysis

Powered by Confident Cannabis
1 of 5

Global Cannabinoids
6445 S Tenaya Way
NV 89113
formulation@globalcannabinoids.io
(805) 210-6402
Lic. #74911

Sample: 1907NVC1046-4636
Strain: n/a
Batch #: BZD190712; Lot #: 2390;
Sample Received: 07/15/2019; Report Created: 07/18/2019

Broad Spectrum Zero-THC Distillate BZD190712
Concentrates & Extracts, Distillate, Other
Harvest Process Lot: ; METRC Batch: ; METRC Sample:

	THCa	Total THC	Total CBD
	<LOQ	<LOQ	95.726%

Cannabinoids

Analyte	LOQ %	Mass %	Mass mg/g	
THCa	0.048	<LOQ	<LOQ	
Δ9-THC	0.048	<LOQ	<LOQ	
CBDa	0.048	0.826	8.26	
CBD	0.481	95.002	950.02	
CBC	0.024	1.405	14.05	
CBG	0.024	0.215	2.15	
CBN	0.048	0.657	6.57	
THCV	0.024	<LOQ	<LOQ	
Δ8-THC	0.024	<LOQ	<LOQ	
CBGa	0.024	<LOQ	<LOQ	
CBDV	0.024	0.330	3.30	
Total		98.435	984.35	

Notes:

Total THC = THCa * 0.877 + Δ9-THC + Δ8-THC
Total CBD = CBDa * 0.877 + CBD
LOQ = Limit of Quantitation; The reported result is based on a sample weight with the applicable moisture content for that sample; Unless otherwise stated all quality control samples performed within specifications established by the Laboratory. Cannabinoids analyzed by SOP-021.

6631 Schuster Street
Las Vegas, NV
702) 826-2700
http://www.nvcann.com

Hui Wang
Hui Wang
Scientific Director

Confident Cannabis
All Rights Reserved
support@confidentcannabis.com
(866) 506-5866

All pass limits are as specified in NAC 453.A and DPBH Policies. Unless otherwise stated all quality control samples performed within specifications established by the Laboratory. This product has been tested by NV Cann Labs using valid testing methodologies and a quality system as required by Nevada state law. Values reported relate only to the product tested. NV Cann Labs makes no claims as to the efficacy, safety or other risks associated with any detected or non-detected levels of any compounds reported herein. This Certificate shall not be reproduced except in full, without the written approval of NV Cann Labs. Uncertainty information is available upon request. All analysis were performed at NV Cann Labs unless otherwise stated. Sampling Plan SOP-001 and Sampling Method SOP-027 were used to collect samples. If sample(s) are NOT collected by NV Cann Labs, result(s) apply to the samples as received.

Certificate of Analysis

Powered by Confident Cannabis
1 of 1

Global Cannabinoids
6445 S Tenaya Way
NV 89113
formulation@globalcannabinoids.io
(904) 312-1834
Lic. #74911

Sample: 1909NVC1438-7359
Strain: n/a
Sample Received: 09/16/2019; Report Created: 09/19/2019

CBD gummies 20mg Zero-THC
Ingestible, Soft Chew, Other
Harvest Process Lot: ; METRC Batch: ; METRC Sample:

	THCa	Δ9-THC	CBD
	<LOQ	<LOQ	19.920 mg/unit

Cannabinoids

Analyte	LOQ mg/unit	Mass mg/unit	Mass mg/g	
THCa	0.120	<LOQ	<LOQ	
Δ9-THC	0.120	<LOQ	<LOQ	
CBDa	0.120	<LOQ	<LOQ	
CBD	0.120	19.920	4.980	
CBC	0.060	<LOQ	<LOQ	
CBG	0.060	<LOQ	<LOQ	
CBN	0.120	<LOQ	<LOQ	
THCV	0.060	<LOQ	<LOQ	
Δ8-THC	0.060	<LOQ	<LOQ	
CBGa	0.060	<LOQ	<LOQ	
CBDV	0.060	0.080	0.020	
Total		20.000	5.000	

1 Unit = Gummy, 4g
Notes:

Total THC = THCa * 0.877 + Δ9-THC + Δ8-THC
Total CBD = CBDa * 0.877 + CBD
LOQ = Limit of Quantitation; The reported result is based on a sample weight with the applicable moisture content for that sample; Unless otherwise stated all quality control samples performed within specifications established by the Laboratory. Cannabinoids analyzed by SOP-021.

6631 Schuster Street
Las Vegas, NV
702) 826-2700
http://www.nvcann.com

Brenda Shalloo
Brenda Shalloo
Scientific Operations Director

Confident Cannabis
All Rights Reserved
support@confidentcannabis.com
(866) 506-5866

All pass limits are as specified in NAC 453.A and Taxation Department Second Policies. Unless otherwise stated all quality control samples performed within specifications established by the Laboratory. This product has been tested by NV Cann Labs using valid testing methodologies and a quality system as required by Nevada state law. Values reported relate only to the product tested. NV Cann Labs makes no claims as to the efficacy, safety or other risks associated with any detected or non-detected levels of any compounds reported herein. This Certificate shall not be reproduced except in full, without the written approval of NV Cann Labs. Uncertainty and statement of conformity are available upon request. All analysis were performed at NV Cann Labs unless otherwise stated. Sampling Plan SOP-001 and Sampling Method SOP-027 were used to collect samples. If sample(s) are NOT collected by NV Cann Labs, result(s) apply to the samples as received.

I hope that when you've finished this chapter, you will have a good base of knowledge as to how you can get started with CBD, and some inkling of what the next steps are that you may want to take.

But just to make things interesting, I will also, here, present you with a warning: that I am—to some extent—a sailor making weather forecasts in the middle of a maelstrom. Each day, companies are bringing forth new CBD products—mine included—and consumers are providing feedback about what they like and don't like. At the same time, new research is telling us about areas where CBD has once again been proven to be useful. Each month that goes by, we know a little more than we did the month before. So I'll do my best. I'll let you know how I think we ought to steer the ship.

But—in keeping with the maritime analogy—I hope you'll take everything with the smallest grain of salt, too.

* * *

When it comes to getting started with CBD, there's a broad spectrum of delivery methods available to consumers. I think it is important that the reader become familiar with these, so they can select the most effective product for themselves. CBD can be taken as a pill. It can be mixed with a carrier oil when used for tincture formulations. It can be absorbed topically. It can be mixed into a food and eaten as an "edible." Almost any food can be infused with CBD. (You've no doubt already noticed how many juice bars and smoothie stands offer to

add CBD to your drink for a small upcharge.) It can be smoked or vaped. There are lollipops and lotions. There are even CBD bath bombs!

That makes CBD kind of unique. It also asks consumers to make more choices.

Many of the compounds, supplements, and medicines that Americans take tend to be confined to one established delivery mechanism. Let's take aspirin as an example. When most people want to take aspirin to relieve pain or reduce a fever, they swallow a pill. There are chewable, flavored aspirins for children, and some aspirin-based topical creams, but most people are thinking of swallowing a capsule when they require the benefits of aspirin.

Then, to take a contrasting example, let's look at menthol decongestants. Most of the time these are going to be deployed in creams that consumers rub on their chests or under

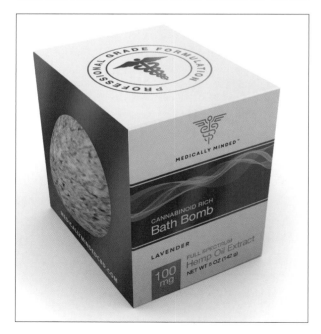

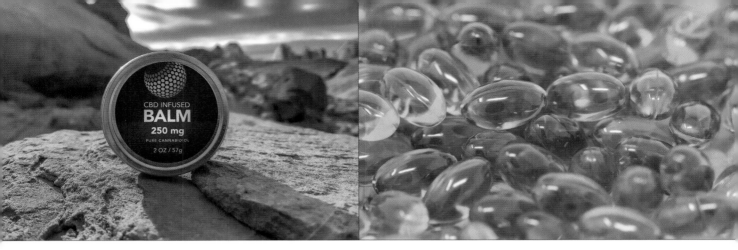

Full Spectrum Hemp softgels gathered in bulk and ready for testing and packaging.

their noses. There are also menthol cough drops that can help reduce congestion . . . but nobody drinks a menthol smoothie!

My point is, when consumers walk into a drugstore to purchase aspirin or menthol, they have a pretty good idea of how it's going to be delivered to them. Years and years of history, customer satisfaction data, and sales numbers at the register have told retailers and manufacturers how consumers prefer to take aspirin and menthol.

But one of the challenges we have—living now, in the exciting early days of CBD—is that we don't have years of data. Companies like mine are still learning the ways in which customers would like to use CBD. This is not necessarily a bad thing. Manufacturers are able to meet customer demand in this area—not least because CBD is able to be delivered in a vast variety of ways. People can have fun and be creative with it, adding it to foods and beverages and making it a delicious experience. I think these are good things.

However, the only potential challenge is that it's hard to tell someone new to CBD the way they should be expected to take it. There are no expectations. There are trends, but they change. The wide range of CBD delivery possibilities can leave people feeling paralyzed by choice.

One reason that the delivery mechanisms for CBD are ever-evolving is that CBD's status itself is evolving in our consciousness.

Is CBD a supplement? Is it a medicine? Is it a health food? Is it an ingredient?

I would argue that the answer to all of these questions is "Yes!"

My personal suspicion—because of CBD's unique status and properties—is that in a few years, we're going to view it a little like exercise.

For example, is exercise medicine? It certainly can be. Physicians can prescribe exercise for people who need it. Exercise, like CBD, is also something that would benefit most people if they did it. Studies have continued to show that there is virtually no downside to either exercise or CBD and that the vast majority of people only see positive gains.

I'd be remiss if I didn't also include that many people exercise simply because it makes them feel good and can be fun, and that's OK, too! Many people are involved in CBD simply because they like the way that it makes them feel. They may not have a specific illness or

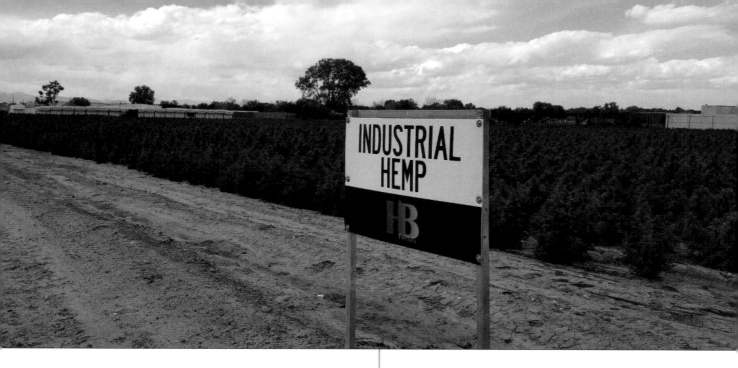

condition they are trying to treat, but they've noticed that they just feel better after using CBD. Which absolutely makes sense scientifically when you consider the way the endocannabinoid system sort of "runs the show." Others enjoy the culture of CBD and find that it fits into their larger culture of natural medicine, meditation, self-improvement, and self-knowledge. They see it as an asset in their journey to being the best they can be.

So, in conclusion, if you're reading this book and you're new to hemp cannabinoids and CBD specifically, I totally understand the frustrations you may feel when faced with so many choices that go along with questions that you feel you may not receive an unbiased answer to. Questions like "What's the right way to use CBD?" and "What's the best way to use CBD?" These are queries this book will attempt to answer. But I want to caution that it's a little like asking, "What's the best way to exercise?" There are lots of ways to exercise. Everything is personal, and while you can look around for examples to follow, eventually you're going to want to find a workout routine and supplementation that feels the best for you personally, because no one body is exactly the same as another.

The good news is that you aren't alone. Many people are on this journey together. As CBD users continue to share their stories—and share the best practices that work for them personally—as the research grows more and more conclusive, consumers will have trail-guides with guideposts to show them their own way, on the American hemp journey.

HOW IS CBD MADE?

So, first things first . . . how does the hemp that is now being legally harvested by farmers across the United States become the CBD products we see on the shelves today?

It's a good question. The short answer is that the CBD is extracted from the hemp plant in concentrated form, and then mixed with a variety of other substances to create the products we know and love. Yet even if you're incurious about the "science side" of how hemp becomes CBD, I'd encourage you to learn a little more about how CBD is extracted from the plant. In the end, it may help you to select a better, safer, and more effective product.

The longer answer is that extraction happens when the cannabinoids are removed from hemp by one of two means: mechanical or chemical extraction. In addition to extracting CBD, these processes can extract other beneficial substances from hemp like terpenes. People who are making a CBD extraction (or any other kind of cannabinoid extraction) are thinking, "What do I keep in, and what do I leave out?" This balance of inclusion and exclusion will determine the final character of the product.

The first method is mechanical extraction. In CBD packaging, you will also sometimes see this method called "solvent-free extraction." It simply means that CBD-containing resins

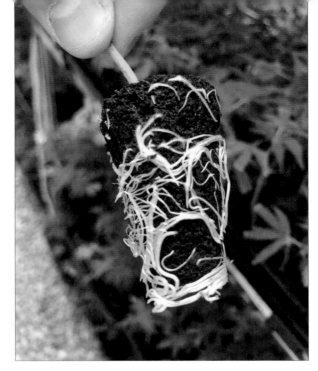

Every gardener knows how important root structure is to the health of the plant, and our experienced farmers are no different.

from the hemp plant have been physically removed and concentrated together. This can be done by using a pressurized carbon dioxide pump to break down the hemp and cause the CBD to be separated. (This is probably the most expensive method of CBD extraction for producers.) Another common mechanical

LEFT: Strain selection and the breeding of hemp genetics allow our farmers to increase naturally occurring cannabinoids. RIGHT: Smaller farms across the USA, using old-school curing methods, are benefiting from a booming industry by supplying local shops and business owners.

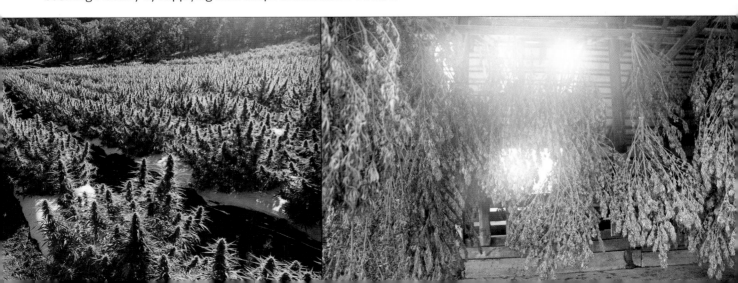

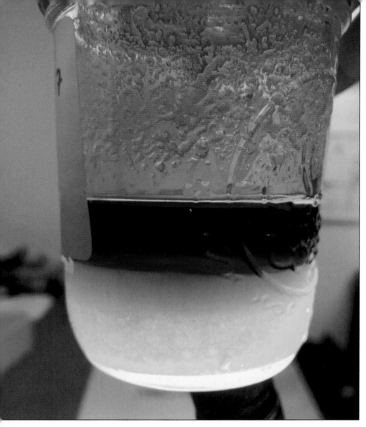

Hemp flowers are frozen as soon as they are cut to preserve the terpenes and then extracted while frozen to retain the full plant profile as pictured in this Hemp CBD Live Resin.

method is using steam to separate the CBD by boiling the hemp (in a series of glass tubes that look very similar to a bootlegger's still) and collecting heated oil vapor that contains the concentrated CBD. Because it does not use chemicals, many health-conscious CBD users favor a product that has been extracted mechanically.

The other method of extraction is chemical extraction, sometimes called "solvent extraction." This involves adding a complex mix of alcohol, butane, or hexane to hemp plant materials in order to strip the CBD out of the plant. As with mechanical extraction, those who employ chemical extraction find that by fine-tuning their process, they can also change the extent to which compounds other that CBD will also be extracted from the hemp. After the chemical extraction is complete, any remaining solvents are removed from the CBD. Ideally, only trace amounts (or no amount) will remain. Because of how it works, some consumers have raised concerns about the safety of chemical extraction. The chief concern is generally that a harmful amount of the extraction chemical will remain in the finished CBD product. This has especially been voiced regarding chemically extracted CBD made in countries with weak laws governing food and drug safety.

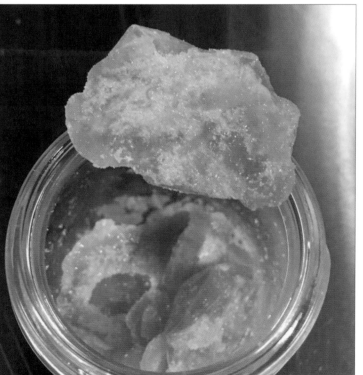

The first THC free terpene infused CBD Isolate "terpsolate" made for dabbing.

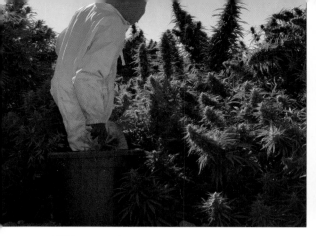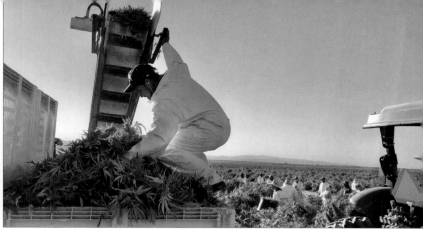

LEFT: Hemp fields need regular weeding and trimming as they grow, so that all flowering buds have access to the nutrients the sun provides. RIGHT: Loading hemp onto shoots for transportation is sticky work, so workers are equipped with suits and gloves in order to preserve trichomes and terpenes glowing on the surface of the buds.

Once the CBD has been extracted—either mechanically or chemically—the concentrate can then be added to a wide variety of products for consumers to use. For some products, such as those containing the highest levels of CBD, the concentrate is further refined into distillates. A distillate is generally defined as a 99 percent pure CBD concentrate. It is typically used in products like tinctures, and in softgel medicines that need to be extremely strong. (More about these examples later.)

As we will see in this chapter, CBD is a remarkably versatile substance when it comes to its healing properties. I think we are doubly lucky that CBD is also versatile when it comes to the way it can be incorporated into almost any physical delivery device. Because of the malleability of CBD concentrate, we can find ways to apply it all across the board. I think that this will help us to bolster its power as an agent of healing.

HOW MUCH TO START WITH?

The specifics of how much CBD someone should start with is probably one of the things people new to CBD ask about the most. I'll answer that question in two ways, a short way and a long way.

Because I hate holding people in suspense, here's the short way: Start small. Especially if you have never activated your endocannabinoid system before. I'm not gonna ask you if you've ever smoked a doobie with your buddies in high school but . . . if you have taken a "hemp cannabinoid product" before, you could start with more. If you're an adult of average size, start with 10mg per day. Take it at bedtime. Make a note of how it affects you— keep a log or journal if you like—and only consider increasing the dose after a few weeks. Everyone I have ever spoken to said that it was the best night's sleep they've had in a long time. However, there are other things to pay attention to, as well. If you usually have pain when rising in the morning, was it alleviated at all? If you are usually swollen in the feet or have stiffness in your legs or hands, was that slightly less of an annoyance? Honestly, if you felt *no* difference at all, you definitely need to increase the dosage for the following evening. Hemp creates what's called a "bell-shaped" curve in the body, so taking too much isn't really possible. The body will discard what it

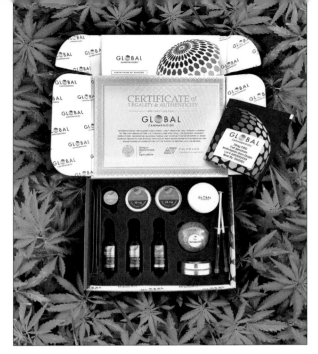

A sample box is the perfect way for businesses to find their niche in the hemp community with a variety of delivery methods catering to customer preference.

does not use. However, once the endocannabinoid system has been activated, and begins to seek out ways to realign the body, you may suddenly feel like taking an extra drop . . . or three . . . one night, which wouldn't be such a bad idea. Listen to your body, at all times. You will be surprised at the ways it will speak to you about its needs, once you begin a hemp regime. Whether that is just a CBD product or a Full Spectrum tincture.

The first thing to keep in mind is that we have evidence that CBD does *not* impact everyone identically. We know that a few people will experience side effects, but most will not. We also know that CBD will impact each person's endocannabinoid system differently; each person has a unique endocannabinoid tone. Some people will get a stronger response from CBD than others, and no two people will experience CBD's effects in exactly the same way. Thus, keep in mind that when your friend tells you they found the "perfect dose" of CBD, it may be the perfect dose for them, but not for you.

Many people make their CBD dosing about finding the lowest amount of CBD that still "does the job." Why is this the case? Well, unless you're in the small minority that experiences side effects, there's no health-related reason to want to take less CBD. It continues to be a very safe substance. However, it is possible for the physical issues that CBD treats to become more severe over time. Because of this, keeping a base dose of CBD low can "give you somewhere to go" if increased pain calls for increasing amounts of CBD.

The next thing to consider when it comes to dosing is the reason why you are taking CBD. As we have seen, much of the research is still new. However, differences in the amounts of CBD used to treat certain conditions are beginning to emerge. For example, we have seen that neurological conditions like epilepsy (again, let me say that you should be working with a physician if you have epilepsy) require large amounts of CBD; it is often prescribed to epileptics at a rate of hundreds of milligrams per day. At the other end of the spectrum are the many people who take CBD for occasional sleeplessness and mild nervousness. For these folks, 10mg (or even less) often does the trick. Some of them don't even need to take it regularly and only use it when they have a bout of sleeplessness or nerves . . . and it's still effective.

It can also change things if you are taking CBD to address a condition confined to a certain part of the body. As we saw in the chapter on medical conditions, topical application of CBD has been shown to eliminate excessively oily skin in clinical studies. Will taking CBD orally *also* help fix oily skin? It may, but those results are not as clear. Based on what we know now, you would probably want to go with a topical application. Likewise, if you take CBD for pain in a certain body part, a localized external application might be the most effective way to go.

Despite CBD's astounding record of being virtually free of serious side effects, it is always a good idea to start slowly with any substance you're consuming for the first time. Whether it's a new spice in food or a new substance with medicinal properties, you don't want to use too much the first time. For this reason—as I noted in the short version above—most people find that beginning with 5mg is a good place to start. It's recommended that most users take their first 5mg at bedtime, simply because one of the rare side effects can be sleepiness. (Note that sleepiness and greater ease falling asleep when you're already tired are two separate things.) If CBD doesn't make you immediately sleepy, you can then start taking it any time of day that you like.

If you live in a state where THC is legal, you will also have the option of trying CBD products that also contain THC. As we've seen in our examination of using cannabinoids to treat different medical conditions, there are a few examples of treatments that combine CBD and THC working very well. If you think that a product containing both CBD and THC would be most effective for you, then you will want to educate yourself on the ratios you will see on the packaging of products containing both CBD and THC. Generally, the product will show the ratio first, and then the ingredients. For example, a product label might read:

8:1, CBD: THC

This package is telling you that it contains eight parts CBD for every one part THC. Many of these products that combine CBD and THC contain very small proportions of THC. Configurations such as 1:24 CBD: THC and 1:20 CBD:THC are not uncommon. However, options with 1:1 CBD:THC are also available. As you would with CBD alone, you'll want to experiment to find the dosage that suits you best. It is always important to remember that THC can cause impairment in ways that CBD cannot. Everyone's body reacts differently to THC, just as with CBD. When you are just starting out—especially if you are new to THC—I would strongly advise you to begin with a weaker THC content—such as 1:24 CBD:THC—and then increase the amount of THC in your ratio as your learn how your body responds.

When you discuss the amount of CBD you are taking with others in the cannabinoid community, you may hear people use the term "self-titration" when telling the story of their own journey to the correct amount of CBD. There's no need to be confused. "Self-titration" is just a fancy term for tuning and adjusting the amount of CBD you take until you find the "sweet spot" in your dosing. I bring this up because talking to people about their own journey can be a useful way to guide your own. And when you speak with other CBD users, you will also learn that, for some of them, self-titration extends beyond dosing. That is to say, they may find that they prefer one brand of provider to another because of the variant of hemp they use to make their CBD. You'll also hear people who adjust or combine delivery methods for CBD. Others will say that their mood can enter into it. For example: "When I'm feeling low and depressed, I find that using a tincture of CBD helps me most, but when I'm feeling better and I just want to maintain that, I prefer using a vaporizer." In communities where CBD is legal, you will probably also encounter some folks who like to use only CBD in some situations, but a CBD:THC combination for flare-ups of others.

Another term you will hear people in the cannabinoid community use is "microdosing." This simply refers to taking a very small amount of CBD. Microdosing is sometimes encouraged for people who are not taking CBD to address a specific ailment but just want to stay healthy and feeling good. Usually, people who microdose take between 2mg and 5mg of CBD per day. I think that microdosing is a fine approach to CBD, and many people swear by it. However, I want to say one thing about it, which is that you should not allow the name to influence your own journey with CBD. It's all relative. If you are a physically smaller person, taking 5mg for you might be like taking 15mg for someone else. And every endocannabinoid system is different. If yours if very sensitive, you'll just need less CBD to get the job done. So there's no need to feel that you are somehow "micro" or "less than" if you get good results from a very small dose. Do what feels right for you and don't worry about labels.

A final note on dosing is that it's always a good idea to talk to your doctor as you begin your journey with CBD. If you currently take medication that might interact with CBD, talking to your doctor is essential. More and more physicians are becoming familiar with CBD, so you shouldn't be shy about speaking with them. In addition, if your doctor doesn't know much about CBD yet, there's no need to fret. They will be able to educate themselves and/or refer you to colleagues who can advise you on CBD. If you want to see a physician who you're certain will be CBD-literate, you can access online databases maintained by organizations like the Society of Cannabis Clinicians.

FINDING A QUALITY PRODUCT

Like anyone entering a new world of products and services, people who begin using CBD want to ensure that they are getting a high-quality, safe product. In order to achieve this, it's important to get educated about the product and brands you might purchase. Virtually no reputable vendor would ever sell a

CBD product that was dangerous. However, it is possible for certain products to be more effective than others, and marketers of lower-quality products do sometimes become temporarily prevalent. In this connection, here's a quick guide to things to look for (and things to avoid) when evaluating CBD products:

- **Avoid any product with packaging that makes wild claims.** For example, any CBD product that promises to cure all cancers should not be purchased. This is one of the surest signs that you are dealing with an unprofessional, fly-by-night, or law-breaking CBD manufacturer. Not only do over-the-top claims cause great disappointment and suffering for potential CBD users, they hurt the entire industry's reputation. (Wild claims are really frustrating for CBD proponents like myself who want to do things the honest, research-based way. CBD has already been shown to do so many wonderful things, and studies have shown it can have potential cancer-fighting properties, such as the capacity to reduce tumor formation and size. It is totally unnecessary for a manufacturer to make exaggerated claims that hemp cures all cancers, for example, because what it genuinely does is already impressive.) Finally, I implore you to avoid CBD sold with exaggerated claims because the claims are illegal, and people who are willing to do one illegal thing (break FDA packaging laws) might be willing to do another (like provide an unsafe product). Stay far away. With that being said, we (businesses included) can all talk about the POTENTIAL for hemp cannabinoids in various disease processes. It's not a crime to say something "may help with" or "history shows us that" or "future research may prove" because, let's face it, there are lots of plant medicines that can be helpful and even curative to some folks, such as chamomile, lavender, or elderberry. We know these things, and yes, there is research to back it up, but FDA guidelines will shut down companies making outrageous claims.

- **Use products with a strong reputation for independently verified CBD content.** Products manufactured by disreputable companies sometimes mislabel the amount of CBD that the products contain. These mislabeled products can contain more CBD than the label claims, less, or sometimes none at all! For example, a study posted on the FDA website titled "Content vs. Label Claim: a Survey of CBD Content in Commercially Available Products" tested the content of twenty-five CBD products available over the counter in Mississippi. It found that only one of twenty-five represented the amount of CBD it contained with perfect accuracy. Some products were slightly off (one product claimed to contain 500mg of CBD but contained 521mg), and some were drastically off (another claimed to have 200mg of CBD but when tested contained only 10mg). Three of the twenty-five products contained no CBD at all! Another study of CBD labeling accuracy was published in the *Journal of the American Medical Association* in 2017 that tested the labeling accuracy of CBD products ordered through the web. About 70 percent did not contain the amount of CBD that was indicated on the packaging. If you are buying a CBD product in a brick-and-mortar store, it's a great idea to chat with the vendor and ask how they ensure the labels on the products they stock are accurate. (A trustworthy vendor will not mind being asked this question.) If you are ordering CBD over the Internet, it's good to do your own research about any brands that are unproven or unknown to you. Remember, authentic, high-quality producers of pharmaceutical-grade CBD will have nothing to hide. The absolute best way to make sure the product you want is the product you

think it is is to ask for a lab report on their "finished product," meaning the actual product you are holding in your hands. The finished product lab report is truly the tell-all. The best companies will have a QR code on the package so you can pull up the lab report by scanning the QR code. All finished products have a batch number or lot number to refer to, so you can see EXACTLY what's in the package you are holding. No company should be without a third-party lab report on their finished product. It should be a third-party reputable lab report that is well versed in how to deal with hemp cannabinoids. Remember that this industry is just starting out, and the equipment needed to truly read and deliver an accurate report is complex and expensive. If someone is trying to sell you a product with what seems to be a "too-good-to-be-true" CBD content, and their lab report is from ABC Laboratories in Nowhere Town . . . well. You may want to chat with some other folks before buying. Don't be afraid to ask lots of questions and understand the terminology being thrown at you. Believe it or not, there are a lot of people selling hemp who don't know a thing about it. Within a few minutes you should have a good feel of the seller's knowledge base and know if you need to shop on or not. Ask if they've tried it. How long they have been selling for. The response they get. After reading this book, you should have a good grasp of what is what, so don't let someone talk down to you. That's not hemp culture. Number one thing to guide you, though, is do not buy from someone who cannot provide you with a third-party lab report. Think about it like this . . . If they can't show you what is in their product, do they even know what is in their product?

- **Trust your gut when it comes to the growing and manufacturing processes.** The conditions in which the hemp plants used to produce CBD are grown can be very important to some consumers. Many people who use CBD are passionate about organics, for example, and would prefer that any product that enters their body be grown organically. There may certainly be something to this point of view. We know that soil conditions can have a large influence on the quality of plants. Metals in the soil or similar contaminants can find their way into the final plant product and end up in the person who consumes the plant. In addition to the soil itself, the processes used to harvest hemp and extract the CBD can have an effect on the product, as

well. For example, CBD extractions that are done imperfectly can leave behind more-than-trace elements of potentially dangerous solvents. What to do about all this? Well, if you're a person who feels strongly about organics, then you'll want to check the packaging. Most CBD products that are organically grown say so. Looking for CBD from "American-made" hemp is also a good way to help ensure a safe, high-quality product. (If your CBD comes from hemp grown outside of the United States, find out where. If it's from a country with lax—or nonexistent—regulations about soil quality and pesticides, you may want to rethink your choice of brands.) And if you have questions about the manufacturing and extraction processes used by a particular producer, don't be afraid to look for information on their website. Any quality manufacturer will be proud to discuss the extraction process they use.

- **Don't buy a product that plays coy about whether or not it actually contains CBD.** You generally won't find these in reputable stores that specialize in cannabinoids, but there are products aimed at the CBD consumer that use evasive packaging to merely hint that they contain CBD. Well, here's a spoiler. About 99 percent of them are hinting because they don't actually contain any CBD! Or they contain such a minimal amount that they cannot specify the proper strength. Taking raw hemp oil and adding it to a "carrier" oil like MCT(coconut), hemp seed, or olive oil is how differing milligram (mg) strengths are created . . . so they could be totally misleading you about the ratio of cannabinoid-rich hemp oil and carrier oil. Make sure the packaging states 500mg or 1000mg. You should then be able to see how much is in each dose by reading the label on the back. This is also important to take note of, as this amount will vary. I have seen some tincture bottles that are 500mg, with only 5mg of CBD per dose. Others can go up to 8mg per dose. This is important information for you! In other words, a company should always know and be able to clearly state what is in their product. Sometimes, shady folk sell these products that use "weasel words" such as "contains 100 percent pure hemp extract" on their packaging. Now, that could mean the product contains CBD, but it could also mean it contains THC, CBDA, or even basic hemp seed oil, which contains no cannabinoids at all. At the end of the day, you have no way of knowing. And the reason the manufacturer doesn't want you to know is very likely because you won't like the answer. Don't put anything in your body if you don't know exactly what it is. A company who can pay the money for laboratory reports more than likely can afford to hire informed, competent teams to design and translate accurate information on their product packaging. If they can't even make clear if their product contains CBD or not, it's a sign that something is likely to be rotten in Denmark.

In conclusion, you want to use the same kind of common sense when purchasing CBD products that you'd use when purchasing anything else that you plan to put in your body. Reputation is important, and so is an openness about the way business is done. The more a CBD company is willing to share its manufacturing processes, the better your odds of being able to trust the product they make. When a company acts like it has something to hide . . . well, there may be a reason for that. You ought to look closer.

CBD OIL

If you didn't skip my section on Rick Simpson, you'll know that oil has been one of the primary delivery vehicles for cannabinoids back to the earliest inklings of cannabis culture in the United States. Oil is one of the first ways that many people encounter cannabinoids,

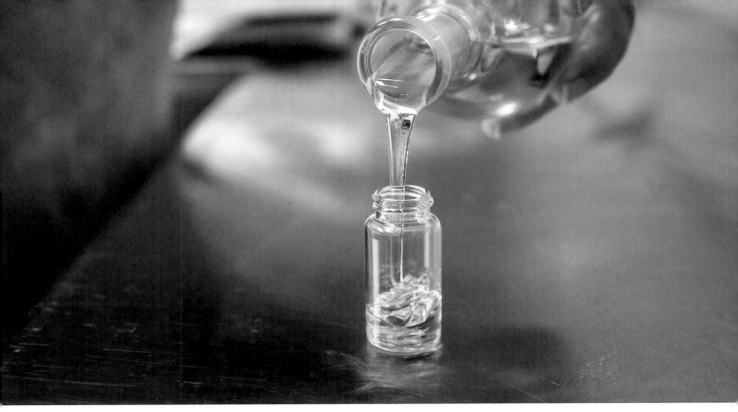

Production teams prepare full spectrum distillate for laboratory testing.

and it can also be an excellent choice of people beginning a journey with CBD.

The first and foremost thing to keep in mind is that "CBD oil" is not "hemp oil" or "Rick Simpson Oil." Hemp oil is generally made with whole hemp plants and will contain both CBD and THC in varying degrees. What matters after this fact is the way it is processed, cured, and handled. The process in which it is manufactured can be, to put it in simplest forms, a matter of differing levels of distillation and the amount of chemical changes. If a product claims to have zero THC and can prove it with a lab report, you have a very high level of processed hemp cannabinoids. There are tinctures available that are "whole hemp extracts," meaning they may not have gone through distillation at all and contain a variety of cannabinoids, including terpenes and some

THC. If you are purchasing a product that claims to be CBD only, the label should clearly state that. You don't have to be an expert in distillation and isolation. Nonetheless, it is important to use common sense. Read the description of what you're purchasing carefully, and if you're making a purchase in a brick-and-mortar store, verify with the clerk that you're indeed buying what the label states you are buying. Don't be afraid to ask questions.

CBD oil is currently exploding in popularity as more people find out about its natural benefits, ease of use, and lack of side effects. It is also popular because it is an easy way to transport CBD in concentrated form. Most people seeking to try CBD for the first time do so via oil or cream. If you are looking to incorporate CBD into your wellness routine, a good rule of thumb is to try a small amount first and see how it impacts you.

Most people who use CBD oil consume it orally. Will you like the taste of it? This tends to vary from person to person. Most producers of CBD oil try to give it a pleasing taste or aftertaste by adding essential oils. Most oils that start as powdered CBD Isolate don't have any flavor to begin with, as it was separated from the rest of the molecular chain, containing all the flavonoids. Despite all that, if the taste of CBD oil does not agree with you, I hope you won't make that the end of your CBD journey. There are many other ways that CBD can interact with the body. Taking CBD orally means that it first has the chance to impact the mouth and stomach, then the digestive system. CBD is metabolized by the liver and will eventually reach your bloodstream (just like any other substance that is metabolized in such a manner). When it comes to the practical "how-to" of taking it orally, that's up to you. As you can see if you watch Rick Simpson's films about his experience, his method of taking hemp oil is to use a needleless syringe-style applicator to put a small amount on his finger. Then he pops his finger into his mouth and sucks or rubs it on his gums. (Again, your style may come down to whether or not you like the taste.)

When deciding on an oral CBD oil, you will also have options related to filtering and carboxylation. Decarboxylated CBD oil has gone through a process that removes a carboxyl group from a molecule, and many believe that the process unlocks the therapeutic processes of the oil. There are also many options for using "raw" nondecarboxylated CBD, too. And because some people believe that both have their own health properties, some vendors even offer a "blend of the two types."

CBD is decarboxylated via a natural process that simply involves heating it. The trick is knowing how high to heat it and for how long. Most of the time, a longer heat at a lower temperature is preferred by purists who like terpenes. Terpenes are what give cannabis its unique aroma and flavor. Some also believe that terpenes are crucial to the therapeutic effects of cannabinoids. Although many consumers never trouble themselves to learn much about it, others hold that decarboxylation is a vital part of the process when it comes to CBD. If you think that it might make a difference for you, I encourage you to educate yourself further on the topic.

SOFTGELS

Softgels are a very popular way to take CBD, and they make monitoring your dosage a snap. A CBD softgel is just what it sounds like—a single dose amount of CBD in a soft capsule-like form that can be swallowed. With capsules, dosing is very exact. Each bottle will let you know how much CBD you can expect to receive within each softgel. Most people take their CBD softgel once to twice a day and make it part of their daily routine.

I think that the appeal of capsules and softgels comes from the fact that American

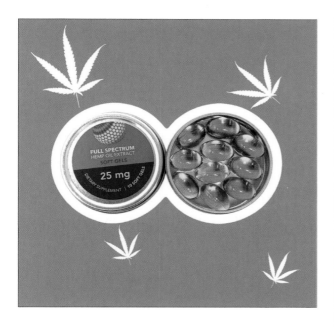

are already very accustomed to "taking pills." There's no equipment to buy, and you can swallow a softgel quite discreetly if you so wish. In addition, an unstudied area of CBD derived from hemp—but one that excites many people—is the possible nutritional benefits to be derived.

As you would with many other nutritional supplements taken in pill form, it's generally better to take a CBD softgel with food. This is because the fatty acids found in many foods can aid in the absorption of the CBD and help digest and deliver it into your bloodstream.

Because there is a considerable connection between the CBD and vegetarian and vegan community, most providers will offer vegan capsule options containing no animal products whatsoever.

What concentration of CBD should you take in a softgel? Many experts in the industry recommend starting with an amount like 10mg and taking it just once a day for several weeks while your body acclimates. After that, you can consider moving to a larger amount in your daily softgel. Most manufacturers make 25mg and 50mg softgels, and some CBD users take one or two of these daily. Getting an idea of how CBD affects you—which I encourage you to do gradually—can help you get a sense of what your optimal dose will be over time.

TINCTURES

Some users of CBD find that taking a tincture works best for them.

"Tincture" is a strange term for many people. It can sound archaic or overly medical. However, there's no need for it to seem so exotic. Technically speaking, a tincture is just anything organic that has been dissolved into a liquid form. Many plants can be made into tinctures. CBD tinctures, or CBD oil, is taken orally. Usually, it is dispensed with an eye dropper. While some people like to use a CBD tincture by adding a few drops to a beverage, the most common method is probably holding it under the tongue until it dissolves. Many fans of CBD tincture hold that this method of taking it allows the mucus membranes under the tongue to absorb the CBD more quickly and effectively. There is large but anecdotal evidence that this has become the preferred method of taking CBD by folks who use it to control seizures. For example, in a 2016 issue of the academic journal *Pharmacotherapy*, researchers from the University

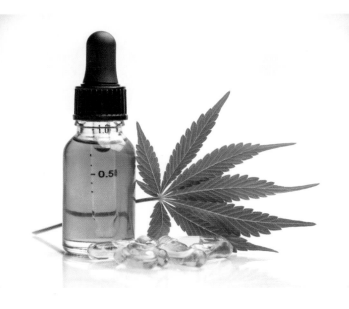

of Mississippi published the study "Current Status and Prospects for Cannabidiol Preparations as New Therapeutic Agents." In this piece, the authors found that there may indeed be a correlation between allowing a CBD tincture to dissolve in this way and overall CBD effectiveness.

Anecdotally, many people also say that a tincture can be one of the quickest ways to get CBD into your system. Therefore, if you're someone who finds that CBD has a fast-acting effect that you like—making you fall asleep or quelling a panic attack, for example—then you may discover that taking CBD via a tincture is your preferred method.

The labeling of CBD tinctures can sometimes initially confuse people, so I should say a word about that. Typically, a bottle of CBD tincture will be labeled with the total amount of CBD the bottle contains—*not* the amount of CBD per drop, or per eye dropper. Many bottles of CBD tincture come in 550mg and 1200mg sizes. Again, this is the amount of CBD *in the entire bottle*. Properly labeled products will tell you how many milligrams you are getting per full dropper.

Tinctures are not outlandishly expensive, but they are often not the cheapest way to enjoy CBD. Tincture bottles come in different sizes and concentrations. Large bottles, such as one-ounce tinctures, with 1000mg of cannabinoids total, can easily go for over $100. Because of this, if you're a first timer, I strongly recommend that you start with a smaller bottle to see how you like it. If it becomes your favorite way of taking CBD, then it can make sense to invest in a larger and potentially pricier container.

VAPING

The fact that CBD is a substance that can be inhaled is allowing it to be enjoyed by the large segment of Americans who already enjoy vaping. For people who vape, switching to a vape canister that contains CBD is a very easy adjustment.

According to recent reporting by Reuters, nearly 11 million Americans vaped or used e-cigarettes in 2018, and that number is on the rise. Vaping is also especially popular with American adults under age thirty-five. Interestingly, we also know that vaping is slightly more popular with men than with women, and—for reasons unknown—it's very popular with the LGBTQ community (approximately 9 percent of LGBTQ Americans enjoy vaping). Vaping is also popular around the world. According to research by Imperial College London and the University of Athens, about 12 percent of EU residents vape. (It is more difficult to estimate the popularity of vaping in Asia. Asia is the largest market globally for tobacco smoking, and many believe that the tobacco industry has intentionally suppressed vaping in many Asian countries, with an eye to keeping the populace using tobacco. For example, Singapore—after what many perceived as tobacco industry lobbying—banned all vaping products in 2018. However, many residents of Singapore continue to vape extralegally.) My point with these statistics is to show that the large, preexisting population of people who already enjoy vaping are ready-made to begin using their hobby to enjoy the benefits of CBD.

Vaping allows a consumer to inhale a small amount of CBD. When it is breathed in, the CBD rests against the interior of the lungs before being absorbed. After absorption, it is diffused into the bloodstream and circulated to the rest of the body. CBD can be vaped from virtually any device. Small personal vape pens can be used discreetly, but consumers can also enjoy a variety of more conspicuous (and, for some, more satisfying) vaporizing devices of all shapes and sizes. CBD can be purchased in vape cartridges. These cartridges will generally have the amount of CBD contained printed on the product labeling so consumers can

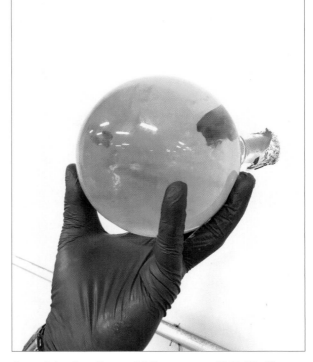

One of the first liters of full spectrum CBD Distillate made from USA-grown hemp.

understand the amount they will be vaping. Just like tinctures—and just like other vape products—vape cartridges can also be flavored to allow consumers to enjoy a pleasant taste while they vape. (Also like tinctures, vaping is more appropriate for consumers who are comfortable with a somewhat approximate dose that may be slightly different every time.)

Vaporizers (or just "vapes") are electrically powered and use heat to turn a liquid (sometimes called "vape juice") into a smoke-like substance that can be easily inhaled. Because they are electronic, vaporizers require a power source. Some of them run on batteries that can be replaced, while many others are rechargeable (many via a USB port).

If you're the type of consumer who is likely to be vaping CBD in the same indoor space each time, then a "tabletop vaporizer" might be the right model for you. These vaporizers are typically larger and stationary and are so named because they can sit on a tabletop near a power source. Many people believe that because tabletop vapes are larger and stronger than portable handheld vaporizers, they tend to deliver a better overall function. Some tabletop vapes feature LED screens that show the temperature of the vape juice being heated or feature a countdown to when they will be ready for use. Tabletop vapes have been around in their current form for over a decade, and they are continuing to grow in popularity. I also strongly recommend a tabletop vaporizer if you're the kind of person who is not shy about your vaping and maybe would even want to make it a conversation piece. A big tabletop model will certainly do the trick when a visitor comes to your home—and you want them to notice your newest lifestyle accoutrement. For some people, a drawback to a tabletop vaporizer is the cost. It's hard to get one for less than $100, and many of the high-end models can close in on a grand. It would probably be a shortsighted idea to invest in a tabletop model if you are new to vaping and unsure if it's something you'll enjoy. However, if you find that it's the way you most enjoy using CBD, then investing in a top-tier model may be the right move.

When it is activated, a vaporizer can heat liquid to over 400 degrees Fahrenheit. However, the vaporized liquid that the consumer breathes in will only be pleasantly warm and will not cause burns. Some vaporizers use a physical element to touch the liquid and make it vaporize, while others simply conduct heat through the liquid. Whichever model or mechanism you select, the effect will be the same. Most vaporizers feature a permanent, attached mouthpiece that the user presses to his or her lips in order to take a draw of the vaporized fluid. However, some also feature tubes or hoses. Consumers can find the make and model they like most when it comes to mouthpieces. The type of mouthpiece used will do little to impact the absorption of CBD.

Vaping is a very popular way for consumers to try CBD for the first time. As I noted at the beginning of this section, vaping has its detractors—many of which, I believe, unfairly conflate safe vape products with illegal and dangerous ones—but the statistics are unerringly firm on vaping's safety compared to any other smoking/inhaling activities. Because of this, many consumers find it a fun and agreeable way of enjoying CBD and other natural health substances with a low-to-negligible risk. Other benefits that may make vaping the right choice for you are that its effects are near-to-immediate. One does not need to dissolve fluid under the tongue for a minute or more for the vaped substance to begin entering the bloodstream. It also allows for consumption nearly everywhere. Vaping also does not "scream" that you are using CBD. Consumers who might like to keep their use of CBD a private choice will be able to vape in public with nobody the wiser.

Are there any reasons why vaping CBD *wouldn't* be the right choice for you? Well, if you're one of the folks who is concerned about the reports that not enough research has been done into the safety of vaporizer use, then remember a panoply of other options for enjoying CBD remain. As I've expressed, my personal belief is that vaping CBD is very safe. However, if you're going to be worried—albeit, in my opinion, unnecessarily—about related health effects, then you should probably go another route. Not because there's any big danger, but because if you're worrying, then you won't enjoy yourself.

There are also reasons why vaping might be for you that have to do with things like your personal style. For one, vaping takes a little bit of patience—not for the CBD to affect you, but to prepare to access the CBD in the first place. You have to wait for your vaporizer to heat up, you have to deal with replacing cartridges, and you have to clean your vaporizer every once in a while. While this might not be too much of a delay in your gratification, it *does* take longer than, say, sticking your finger in a bottle of oil and rubbing it on your gums. Other factors that might make vaping less than ideal would be the things involved in investing in a vaporizer—if you don't want to deal with it, or if the cost would be too prohibitive, then you can go in other directions.

The only other reason I can think of is that you're an outdoorsy type who is going to be away from power outlets (or replacement batteries) for an extended period. If you're looking to enjoy CBD while hiking the Pacific Crest Trail in one go—for example—then you may want to think about another method for taking your CBD.

I think that some people will experiment with CBD in many forms and discover that they like vaping the best. However, I think a vastly larger amount of people who already vape will discover that CBD makes a great addition to their preexisting hobby of vaping. They will be curious about CBD, and vapable CBD will make it easy and fun for them to try. Then they can take advantage of the numerous health benefits CBD has to offer.

EDIBLES

Another way to enjoy CBD is by chewing and eating an edible. "Edible" is sort of a big-tent term for any food product that has been infused with CBD. Like anything eaten, an edible will go to the stomach, where it will be

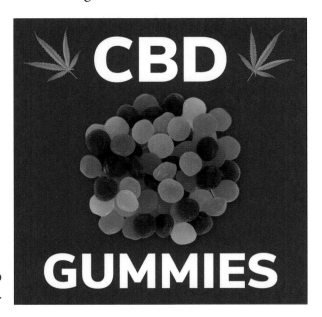

Gummies are a delicious way to incorporate CBD into your daily routine.

digested. The CBD will be processed by the liver and diffused into the bloodstream, where their salutary effects will then begin working.

Consumers will find a wide variety of options for CBD edibles. Some are selected simply because they are fun. A good example would be gummy bears. (An edible like a gummy bear also has the advantage of being a very precise size and so is able to deliver a clear and measured amount of CBD to the user each day.) Other popular edibles include small chewable treats that have also been infused with vitamins and caffeine. An edible like this enables someone to enjoy their morning caffeine, take their morning vitamin, and also take their daily CBD—all at once. I think these can be a great alternative to expensive, artificial, and frequently sugar-filled energy drinks.

Are there benefits and/or drawbacks of CBD edibles? Well, because edibles involve literally subjecting the CBD to your entire digestive system, there are, at least, unique factors involved. Generally, because you are consuming the CBD like a food, edibles mean that it will take at least 30 minutes from the moment of ingestion for the CBD to genuinely absorb into your system. However, there's another side to that coin. Those who report being able to feel a distinct and unique sensation when they take CBD report that using edibles takes long for the effect to kick in, but that the effect "hangs around" longer because of this same mechanism.

The benefit of edibles can also be psychological, and this can help some people stick to a healthy regimen. For many Americans, eating an edible feels like "a treat"—something you do to reward yourself. Something that you don't *have* to do, but that you *get* to do. In contrast, taking a pill or dispensing something from a dropper or syringe can feel like "taking medicine"; it's a "have to" and not a "want to." These kinds of mental maneuvers might sound silly, but they can really make the difference for people who have difficulty remembering to stick to a treatment. If this is you, then perhaps you'll find that edibles are a fun way to take your daily CBD and enjoy all the benefits—without it feeling onerous or boring.

As a final thought, I would be remiss if I didn't point out that when it comes to cannabinoid edibles, THC sort of "got there first." THC edibles have existed on a large scale for many years, whereas CBD edibles are more recent. Thus, when most people in cannabis culture use the single word "edible" by itself, they are probably still referring to THC edibles and *not* CBD. This shouldn't be a problem for you; just make sure to specify "CBD edible" loudly and clearly at the point of purchase. (If you are purchasing your CBD edible at a store that also sells legal THC products, it is a good idea to ask explicitly: "Does this also have THC in it?" Make sure to always read product labeling carefully. With a little common sense and double-checking, you can easily make sure that you're getting the correct kind of cannabinoid in the edible you choose.)

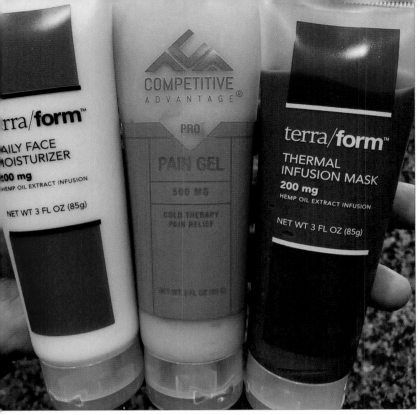

TOPICAL CREAMS AND SALVES

Topicals are another of the most popular ways that consumers are enjoying CBD. As we have seen, CBD is excellent for skincare, and not just the appearance of the skin, but the actual health of it, as well. Whether your goal is to fight acne, make an unpleasant itch go away, or just improve the overall health and appearance of your skin, topically applied CBD can be a powerful and effective tool.

Creams make CBD easy to use. Many people are already accustomed to using a moisturizer or other cream as part of their daily routine, so it's no big stretch for them to incorporate a CBD-based cream, especially when being presented with so much supporting evidence.

Topicals can also be applied to very specific areas of the body. If you've read this far, then you're aware of the remarkable pain- and inflammation-killing properties of CBD—and for this reason, many consumers also like to have a container of CBD cream handy for as-needed applications to certain areas where they may be experiencing pain. This is true even if they already take CBD regularly in another form. For a person dealing with a topical inflammation, for example, or with lower back pain, an application of CBD cream until the symptom subsides can often hit the spot.

CBD cream is made by mixing CBD with a host substance, usually an oil. Like many other topical creams Americans use, CBD creams can be customized and come in different scents or with various consistencies. They can also be made more sensitive for delicate parts of the body. The combination of CBD with specific flowers and herbs added to the creams and salves can be magic when it comes to healing and pain-killing relief.

As a subset of topicals, I'll also include hair shampoos and conditioners. There's a large community of CBD shampoo enthusiasts who swear that the positive impacts of CBD on overall health can be seen and reflected in the hair, especially when applied daily. Like most high-quality shampoos, CBD shampoos are naturally rich in fatty acids and proteins. The unique chemical profile of CBD can also nourish hair. Just as many people have reported remarkable healing effects on cannabinoids on skin, the same is true for hair. Dry, brittle hair that tends to break or crack, and even thinning hair, have all been repaired by CBD. Because so much of the damage our hair endures is natural—such as sun damage or damage from the elements—I think it only makes sense that we turn to a natural source to repair that damage. Some people who like the idea of applying their CBD topically will combine a shampoo with a face cream. I'd encourage you to get creative with it, if you like.

Because they are natural, CBD-based creams and shampoos can also help to combat all the harsh and unnatural things we do to ourselves in the goal of looking great. It's downright shocking the beatings that we give ourselves in the name of appearance. Americans use chemicals on their faces—many literally have "chemical peels"—in the name of looking younger and healthier. They abrade their skin. They use harsh pharmaceutical concoctions to do away with simple blemishes. And none of that includes what they do in order to get gussied up for a particular event. Americans use makeup to make themselves look a certain way temporarily, with no real thought as to how it may impact their skin long term. They put permanent treatments in their hair, style hair with harsh chemicals, or simply brush and comb it until it appears supernaturally straight (or curly).

In short, there's a world of hurt we put onto ourselves in the name of "looking better" in the short term. So what about products that would actually help us "be better"—healthier and happier and feeling better—in the long term? I firmly believe that CBD-based skin and hair products can do both. Moreover, I think something special is going on when people know that the products they're using on their bodies are a healing medicine proven to improve their skin and hair. There's just something psychologically satisfying about that, and it puts us in a healthy frame of mind.

TRANSDERMAL PATCHES

A small percentage of the CBD-using population finds it beneficial to use transdermal patches for getting their CBD intake. A transdermal patch is what it sounds like—a small patch that is placed on the skin. It allows the CBD to be absorbed through the skin into the rest of the body. Transdermal patches don't work as quickly as tincture or a capsule, but your body can start feeling the effects of the CBD in about 15 minutes. Some people prefer transdermal patches because they like the idea of CBD being slowly and steadily absorbed by their body, evenly, over a longer period of time. (Transdermal patches can continue to deliver CBD for up to three hours at a stretch.)

Some people believe that because transdermal patches give the CBD a "starting point" in a very specific spot on the body, they can be more effective for dealing with localized medical issues. Because you use a patch to deliver CBD in order to positively impact your entire body, most manufacturers recommend placing the patch on an area with thin skin, such as the inside of the wrist. However, folks who are passionate about patch placement hold that if their reason for taking CBD is localized, their patch should be, too. In addition, some athletes who use CBD to treat localized injury or soreness report best results from putting a patch directly on the affected area.

It is possible for transdermal patches to deliver CBD in concert with other substances, like THC (or other painkillers). Always make sure that you check the active ingredient list for any patch you purchase.

A final note: many people use patches because they are a discreet way of delivering steady doses of CBD. For example, someone who is going to be "out and about" for the entire day might find it embarrassing to stop and take a capsule every few hours. A patch can be an effective way of privately absorbing a steady stream of CBD with no one the wiser.

BEVERAGES (ALCOHOLIC AND OTHERWISE)

Is there a rule somewhere that CBD can't be fun? If there is, I haven't seen it! Beverages of all sorts containing CBD are hitting the market, and many of them present a fun and safe way for people to try CBD for the first time.

Mixologists across the country are adding CBD to cocktails. CBD won't get you high, so having a cocktail with CBD isn't like having a cocktail with THC. However, we have seen studies showing that CBD can help to ease pain, combat anxiety, and get relief from stress. I don't know about you, but I think all of those things go pretty well with a cocktail at the end of the day.

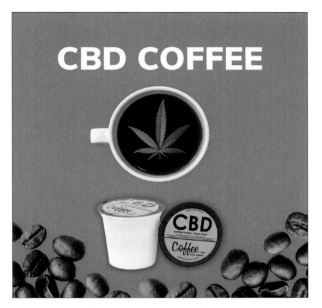

Coffee and CBD are great companions, combining the medicinal benefits of hemp with your morning wake-up routine.

In addition to adding CBD to drinks in restaurants and bars, there is a booming market in bottled and canned drinks containing CBD. Right now, most of the companies producing these beverages are independent, but there are signs that some of the biggest players in the world could get involved. For example, earlier this year, *Inc.* magazine reported that Coca-Cola was in talks with Canadian company Aurora Cannabis to produce a CBD-infused beverage. (Though the formal announcement of the drink has yet to come, shares of Aurora surged 16 percent on the news.) Given the distribution reach of Coca-Cola, a CBD beverage produced, marketed, and sold by them could be a real game changer. And if they do launch such a beverage, there is little doubt that other major brands won't be far behind.

In the meantime, there are already many CBD beverages on the market. Most of them contain 10–30mg of CBD, similar to the amount that most people take as a daily supplement. Many of the beverages available are similar to sodas—they have small amounts of sugar and some flavoring. Others have no sugar at all and go for a profile closer to iced tea. There is CBD coconut water. There is CBD lemonade. There is even CBD cold-brew coffee. One Spanish company is now even marketing a "Cannawine"—red wine infused with CBD. And because many folks just can't get enough of the energy drink format, you better believe there are also CBD drinks marketed to appear as though they were extensions of the high-caffeine drinks that have become so popular with young people.

You can also buy hemp-infused tea that comes in the form of individual tea bags, with the tea inside infused with hemp.

Will all of these drinks stand the test of time? Almost certainly not. I doubt that half of them will still be in the game a decade from now, especially if the larger beverage companies decide to try to muscle them out of the space. But I think they're a fun way in which people can explore CBD. These drinks are certainly not the same way of engaging with CBD as, say, someone who takes a daily supplement. However, lots of folks will try CBD because of these drinks. And I think those people will find that CBD is fun and safe, and even with a single dose it is possible that they'll experience a health effect that they like. These drinks also help to increase the visibility of CBD. Someone who noticed such drinks in the beverage case each time they are at the supermarket is bound to get curious and go online to educate themselves. This is another way CBD beverage can help contribute to the overall understanding of hemp cannabinoids by the public, and help to raise their unique profiles.

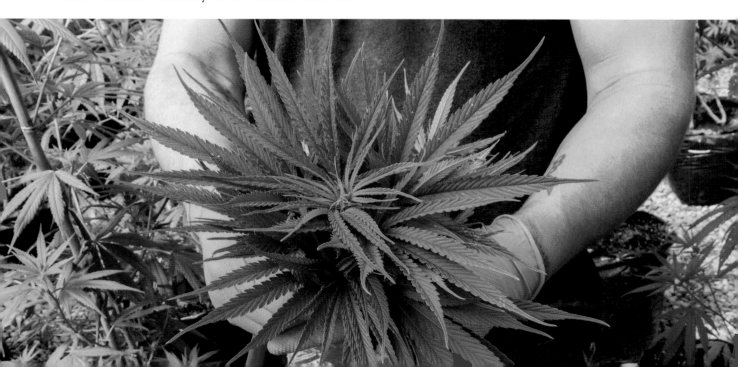

CHAPTER FIVE
WHAT THE FUTURE HOLDS

TRUST AND REGULATION

Trust.

In these early days of CBD, trust is truly the vital currency. It is what people are looking for when they begin to enter this world. Where is a resource I can trust? What is a trustworthy source for information? Who can I trust to deal with me honestly and fairly?

The CBD industry wants regulation, because then everybody wins. A lack of regulation not only means danger to consumers, but leaves open the door for bad actors to spoil the game for everybody.

Consider the trials and tribulations of the vape industry in mid-2019. For years, vaping was on the rise as a vastly safer alternative to tobacco use that offered consumers increased choice. Its acceptance steadily grew. Concern about underage vaping was raised, but politicians were slow to target a product that was demonstrably safer than cigarettes.

Then, quite suddenly, a rash of stories broke in the media about young people who had suffered serious lung conditions and been hospitalized from vaping. The antivaping forces rallied, and legislative bodies across the country began looking seriously at limiting vaping to an additional degree, or even banning it outright. Many consumers who had not educated themselves about vaping could be forgiven for simply thinking: "Hmm, I guess it was more dangerous than we thought."

But only after the damage had been done to vaping's reputation—on a national scale—did the truth come out.

Nearly all of these vaping-related health issues had come about because the victims in question had been using illegal, unregulated vaping products from China, bought on the black market.

And though the vape industry hastened to point out this fact, the black eye was already there. The damage had been done.

Now, when it comes to CBD, there are industry-leading, highly responsible companies going to great lengths to produce pharmaceutical-grade CBD products. (I am proud

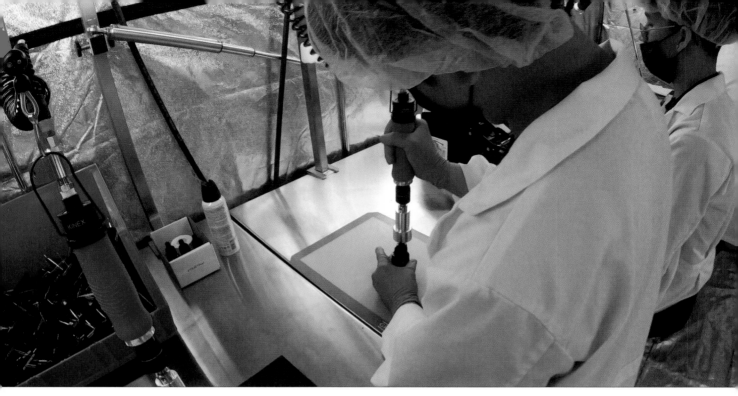

GMP-certified production teams working on assembly for tincture bottles.

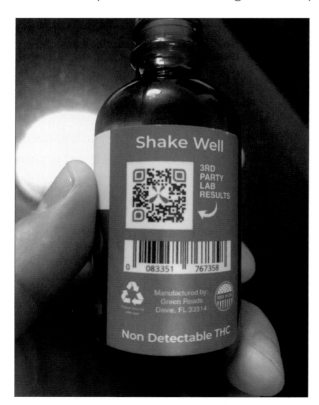

A QR code on hemp tinctures linking to a third-party lab report is exactly what this evolving industry should be doing on every bottle.

to put myself, and every company I'm associated with, in this category.) But let's face it: in every industry, there are people who push second-rate products. There are people who operate without strong ethical integrity. And there are also people who are simply incompetent.

Unfortunately, there are some of these operators in the CBD space.

Just last year, for example, the Centers for Disease Control & Prevention investigated a case in Utah where over fifty people were reported to have experienced symptoms of poisoning after taking a CBD-related product calling itself "Yolo CBD Oil." The CDC investigation showed that the product in question did not contain normal CBD, but rather an illegal synthetic cannabinoid called 4-cyano cumyl-butinaca, which has been known to cause fatalities. In this case, the product misrepresented what it was, and a vendor had sold it as CBD. (Luckily, there were no fatalities in these instances. Authorities were able to raise local awareness and prevent anyone else from purchasing or using the tainted product. And later investigations by the Utah Public Health Laboratory and the Utah Department of Public Safety found that, in actuality, only thirty-four people were actually found to have taken the product.)

The Utah example is an extreme one, because it impacted many people. However, each year, the government tracks tens or hundreds of other cases of poisoning allegedly connected to CBD use. As CBD has exploded in its acceptance and accessibility, these cases have exploded exponentially. According to the American Association of Poison Control Centers, there were three reported instances of human poisonings linked to a CBD product in 2014. In 2015, there were fifteen. In 2016, there were thirty-four. Then the growth gets really exponential. In 2017, there were 118 cases. In 2018, there were 519 cases. And so far in 2019, there have been nearly a thousand.

It's important to note that these are not cases where CBD—or a product claiming to contain CBD—has been *definitely proven* to have poisoned someone. Rather, these are cases alleged to be involved with CBD or CBD-related products.

Some of these cases are going to be psychosomatic based on users trying CBD for the first time. Some of these are going to be the intentional misuse of CBD (by, say, uninformed teenagers who believe they can use it to get "high"). And some of it will be faulty or defective products that do not contain what they claim.

Both vendors and safety-minded consumers should desire the kind of regulation that will help customers understand when they are buying authentic CBD, in which quantities they are buying it, and precisely what the effects will be. (I have the feeling that when this happens, there will be far fewer false positives for "CBD poisoning." People who feel ill will understand that the safe, legal, and well-understood CBD they took is as likely the culprit as an aspirin or a menthol skin cream. Accordingly, they and their physicians will be able to arrive at the *true* cause of the issue more quickly.)

There are other problematic cases where more regulation and standardization would help but that do not involve people claiming to get sick from CBD. Here, I'm referring to cases in which vendors selling CBD—especially online vendors—sell a legitimate CBD product . . . but make such wild speculations about what the product will do that it certainly crosses a line. There are few things more infuriating than when a charlatan claims their cure will *definitely* fix someone's serious ailment, when they know that not to be the case.

A handful of vendors looking to make a quick buck have illegally sold CBD while making unsupported claims of its ability to cure or arrest cancer, heart disease, HIV, and more. Though it has hesitated to act in other ways, the FDA has (thankfully) issued "cease and desist" letters to companies behaving in this manner and in most cases gotten their fraudulent websites taken down.

These unsavory vendors probably do more to hurt the advancement of legitimate CBD than any other factor. While CBD is not a magic cure-all that can always reverse someone's late-stage cancer, it *can* do many remarkable things across a wide array of ailments and health concerns. That's what's so frustrating. With the proper research, there's reason to believe we may see legitimate CBD-based cures and exciting new treatments coming to market in the next few years. Meanwhile, vendors who have sold CBD fraudulently as a "cure-all" create an awareness in the general population that goes like: "People were saying that CBD could 'cure X disease,' but it turned out that that was a lie." When in fact, with the proper research, CBD may indeed cure, treat, or prevent that disease when delivered in the appropriate manner, and in the appropriate amounts. We just don't know. But making consumers close their minds to the possibilities of CBD—before the true research has even been done—is probably the worst thing that we can do.

THE IRREPRESSIBLE POWER OF CBD

When people in the United States want something—especially something that is safe, non-addictive and nonnarcotic—they are going to get it. During alcohol prohibition in this country, well-meaning teetotalers made it illegal—for most Americans, in most circumstances—to have a drink. This resulted in a burgeoning underground rack for illegal booze that was a boon to organized crime and resulted in poisonings from "bathtub gin." When the nation returned to its senses and made consuming alcohol legal again, organized crime was diminished and government regulation made sure that alcoholic beverages were safe to drink.

In another example, Americans seem to greatly enjoy playing the lottery. The fact that the government tried to make lottery games (at least in most states) illegal led to a tremendous source of revenue for organized crime. "Running numbers" and "policy games" created reliable sources of income for criminal syndicates, which could then use these profits to invest in other, more nefarious ventures. But when a movement arose in the 1960s and 1970s to have legal, state-run lotteries administered by the government, consumers showed that they vastly preferred this safe and legal alternative. State and national lotteries soared in popularity, and criminal gangsters lost yet another source of revenue.

Those are both somewhat extreme examples, but I mean to use them to make an important point: I don't think CBD—and perhaps cannabinoids in general—is a force that can be stopped. I think that once Americans understand that it's something they want (and even need), they are going to take the necessary steps in order to get it.

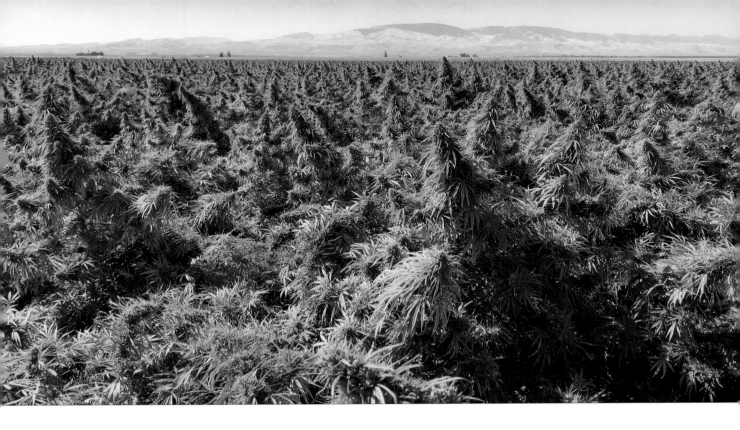

The government can legalize and regulate it to prevent the funding of criminal organizations, or the government can fruitlessly fight an endless battle it can never win.

So far, the arc of things has been in the direction of progress, which heartens me greatly. There is just no reason why CBD and its benefits should not become a general part of our lives and lifestyles.

There's an old saying that sunlight is the best disinfectant. The saying means that openness and honesty is the best policy, as it eliminates the ability of lies, rumors, and misconceptions to grow (like mushrooms in the darkness). I think that's important to remember in terms of what we're trying to do here. There are junctures in history where an opinion or set of beliefs goes from being in the minority to being in the majority. From being something that a small group of people espouses, to being the dominant ideology of the land. From attitudes about technology, to spiritual beliefs, to styles and fashions—it's easy to think of examples where this is true across time. I think that proponents of CBD understand that they have a minority opinion that is closing on the majority day by day. But how best to let that happen? How do we make positive change occur—especially positive change that can lead to vast improvements in the health and well-being of millions of people? I think we do that by making clear that we have nothing to hide. CBD and its helpful properties will speak for themselves. If we're truly confident—which I believe we should be—then we want it to be studied and examined in every way possible.

We want CBD to be held up in the sunlight and examined from every angle, so to speak. If we do that—if we take that attitude at every juncture, one that says, yes, we want every aspect of CBD to be examined with the most rigorous science possible—then it sends a strong message to anybody who still has a shadow of a doubt. It's about confidence. Many of us already know the positive effect CBD has had for ourselves, or for someone who we love. I think that if we can project this confidence, then more and more people who are new to CBD—and who might still have misconceptions about it—are more likely to be impressed. They're more likely to see that in addition to there being a vibrant "cannabis culture" surrounding cannabinoids and their positive effects, CBD advocates are also calling for as much hard science as possible. This is not something pseudoscientific or beyond science. Rather, CBD is something very much of and from the natural realm, simply waiting to be studied.

If we can do that—if we can project this attitude—then it's only a short matter of time until CBD and related cannabinoids get the audience and reach that they truly deserve. We have nothing to fear, and we should act like it. We are excited for all the positive things that the world is going to enjoy once CBD is fully studied and embraced, and I think that excitement can be contagious.

WELLNESS

In the months and years ahead, my earnest hope is that humans as a species continue to make the kinds of change that will help us to focus on creating holistic wellness for ourselves, our neighbors, and our planet. We're living in an age when transformations in technology are making advancements possible that would have seemed like science fiction only a generation ago. We are understanding more about how our own bodies work, and more about how humans work as a species. Yet as I stressed in the opening pages of this book, we are also a species at a turning point.

We are realizing that we cannot continue to live in the way that we have been in the last century. To do so would be ruinous to the ability of our planet to sustain life in the future, and probably to our own ability to be fully happy and actualized creatures. For many years, life expectancy continued to creep ever upward, year after year, as scientific and nutritional advancements taught us more about our bodies and helped us better care for ourselves. But something happened in the 2010s. For the first time in many generations, the average life expectancy in the United States began to go down instead of up. This was especially pronounced in communities of underemployment, disinvestment, and where use of alcohol and prescription opioids were very pronounced.

It seems like experts from every field have strong opinions about why this trend is taking place. Endless "think pieces" have been written. Theories have been bandied about on television news programs.

I think it's important that the root causes of our country's problems be analyzed. But if you ask me, no matter what the ultimate cause—or causes—of this disturbing trend, a few key things will still remain true. Most of the decline in life expectancy is coming from self-destructive things that Americans are doing to themselves. They are seeking out temporary cures that have dire consequences . . . and often fatal side effects. Many Americans are hurting and unhappy. Something needs to be done.

The good news is that some of the smartest people in the country—way smarter than I—are addressing this problem. It's being looked at from every conceivable angle. A holistic approach is being taken to help people. I strongly believe this is the right direction.

I believe that almost all of us can find a way to make the world a better place—whatever we do, and in whatever field we're employed in. We can give a damn, and we can make a difference.

I think it would be almost criminally irresponsible of someone who is an authority on CBD—and what it can do—to stay silent at a time like this.

As we enter the 2020s, vast numbers of Americans need help finding wellness in their lives again. I think most of them are not bad or shortsighted people; they have just lost their way. Anything that can help them take one step back in the direction of health and hope can be meaningful. And the thing about taking one step is that sometimes it leads to another. And then to another. And another.

CBD's scientifically established tendency to help people move away from addictive and self-destructive behavior can be a step in the right direction. People who are abusing opioids or alcohol—or smoking cigarettes, still the number one preventable killer—can use CBD to help break these destructive habits. CBD is relatively inexpensive, and its availability is only increasing. Anybody with an Internet connection can order some. Physicians and counselors who work with people in communities that are struggling with life-shortening vices can be educated about CBD. They can recommend it (in virtually every state, at the time of this writing) without a prescription.

I want CBD to be used as a tool to bring this country back to wellness. I want to look at those charts that show American life expectancy year after year and see that line going back up. Because CBD can be used to address so many issues, I want to help ensure that it *does* address them. The recent blessing by the FDA of CBD to treat epilepsy is a step in the right direction, but it is not enough. Millions of Americans with other medical conditions stand to have their lives improved by CBD, and to have their health boosted significantly, at this very moment, now. At the same time, folks who are struggling with addiction because of a set of dire circumstances that have come to their communities—coupled, it must be said, with the overprescription of opioid medications—need all the help they can get to make a change in their lives. Beating addictions is very difficult to do and often takes multiple tries and approaches. People heading down that hard road can use any asset available. Considering all that they are up against, shouldn't we make sure that CBD is on their side, as well? Something safe, inexpensive, and effective?

I feel passionately about this for the same reason that I got into hemp in the first place. I'm an entrepreneurial person, but I also care about making a difference. I want to leave the world a better place than how I found it. I think there's no question that CBD can make that a very real possibility. This isn't a pipe dream or wishful thinking. As I noted earlier, 40 percent of Americans in their twenties have now tried it. What will it take to get that percentage in other demographics? For people over sixty, the rate is still just 15 percent, yet the elderly are often the most in need of having conditions (like chronic pain) corrected. If it is possible to reach one group, then it is possible to reach another.

I hope it is clear that I intend my tone to be hopeful, not cynical. I firmly believe that Americans are legitimately ready for change and are open to the kinds of possibilities that CBD offers. Historically, cannabinoids have been bifurcated into two categories of use: recreation and medical. However, we are beginning to see a third, as we isolate and examine each one further . . . and that is wellness. CBD products can treat symptoms previously thought untreatable by modern medicine but there is also good evidence that it can cause some diseases and conditions from even happening in the first place. This, in my opinion, is where the new growth

is going to come. It's also the right header for reaching out to some of the people who need help the most. Let's not wait until there is an alcohol or opioid epidemic for CBD to address. Instead, let's work now to help people take a step toward a wellness lifestyle that can hopefully prevent a chronic addiction from occurring in the first place. The more Americans can incorporate CBD into the regular products they use to keep themselves healthy, the better shielded they can be from a whole panoply of challenges.

Psychologists tell us that we are better about making positive changes in our lives when we focus on moving "toward something good" as opposed to "away from something bad"—especially in the long term. Physicians use this when they try to get a person to break a bad habit. For example, cardiologists trying to get a patient to exercise and eat better have long found that using fear—such as portraying in vivid detail the extremely unpleasant heart attack that's likely in a patient's future if they don't mend their ways—can be somewhat effective, but only over the short term. After a few weeks, fear simply ceases to be a motivating factor. However, these same cardiologists find that when they ask patients to imagine all the great things in their future that they wouldn't want to miss—seeing their children graduate from college, getting to hold their grandchildren, and so on—then patients are much more likely to find the strength to make the difficult lifestyle changes necessary.

I think that says something nice about

human psychology and how our brains work. I also think it's the force we can draw upon to help make CBD part of a national wellness movement.

It's my earnest hope that we can help CBD and other beneficial hemp cannabinoids become a vital part of our focus on wellness going forward. I think that when people focus on all the things that a healthy lifestyle that includes CBD will allow them to do, they're more likely to find the strength to commit to positive choices. It's been important that our culture has focused on highlighting the dangers of unhealthy living, opioid abuse, and alcoholism. That needed to be done. But now we need to show people the way out. And we need to give them the best chance of making the exit from unhealthy lifestyles. I believe CBD can be a vital asset for this.

THE FUTURE

You've probably heard the old adage "It's the journey, not the destination." This can be a useful paradigm for so many things in our lives. As we go down the road of life, we're obviously trying to achieve certain things. In the wellness sphere, many of those things will be, no question, health related. We want to look good and feel good. We want to do things that make us proud of ourselves. We want to get a little better every day.

All this activity may result in some ultimate final goal: lowering our blood pressure, fitting into the pants we used to wear in college, etc.

But that final endgame moment will—in the grand scheme of things—be extremely short. What will *not* be short is the trip we take to get there. That will be the vast majority of the journey of our lives.

CBD, like many areas of our lives that concern our well-being, is a journey. In 2019, the first step for many people is hearing about CBD for the first time, and educating themselves about it. I think that many of you are on that part of the journey right now, reading this book. For a majority of you, I believe the next step will be to try incorporating CBD into your own wellness lifestyle.

It's great to have options and choices; consumers love having options in every aspect of their lives. Many people are passionate about their personal style. The neat thing about CBD is that you can take stock of what kind of personality you have when it comes to being ready to engage with CBD and then find a way to work it in. You may want to enjoy the health benefits of CBD, but without making it a large part of your life (and without expending much mental energy dealing with it). In this case, you may want to go for a "set it and forget it" model. Taking a CBD supplement each morning with any other pills, and then enjoying the positive effects—all while giving it no further attention. (Believe me, I understand the appeal of this view. People have only so much bandwidth. Many people have enough going on in their lives that engaging with CBD in this sort of way is the best it's going to get.)

Other people are likely to want to "marinate" in the world of CBD—perhaps literally! For them, CBD will be an endlessly fascinating world with new things to learn and discover around every turn. The kind of consumers who fall into this group may legitimately enjoy each nuance of CBD to be learned and will probably enjoy fine-tuning their intake and the manner in which they take it, many times over.

The analogy that springs to mind is cars. There are some people who just want to know how to put gas in their car, and anything beyond that they'd rather leave to a mechanic. But there are also "do-it-yourself-ers" who enjoy learning everything there is to know about fine-tuning their cars, inside and out.

The great thing about the number of choices available to consumers in the marketplace today is that virtually everybody can be accommodated, no matter what their style.

I also think, as the song goes, we ain't seen nothin' yet!

In the next decade, there will likely emerge new vehicles for CBD that we haven't even considered. Consumers will have the option of more customization than ever before, more kinds of CBD than ever before, and from different sources. As scientific innovations related to CBD also increase, we will see these reflected in mainstream product offerings to consumers. What I would advise consumers of CBD is to watch for such products that are supported by science. (As this craze grows, we may begin to see CBD added to products in such a way that it does not actually do anything. Just as in the late 1800s, electricity was presented as a "cure-all," and in addition to its many useful applications, things were "made electric" that did not need electricity in order to function optimally.) Yet over time, I think we will see any untrue claims about CBD—and unnecessary applications for it—fade away for good. Users will know what they want and will get a true sense of what it actually delivers. And the market will only be richer for it.

I've tried to accomplish a number of things in this book. I've tried to tell the story of how I got interested in CBD. I've tried to profile the researchers doing cutting-edge work on CBD. I've reviewed the medical conditions it can positively impact, and along the way we've seen the stereotypes and regulatory hurdles that CBD faces.

But my larger goal here is trickier. My real motive may not come through clearly from the proceeding pages, so let me just lay it on the line as clearly as I can.

I'd like you to get excited about the possibilities of hemp cannabinoids and CBD specifically, and what it has shown us . . . because I want to make you an advocate for your own health and well-being, as well as the health of the people you care about. Throughout history, we can look at revolutionary medical breakthroughs—which are commonplace today—but that faced resistance in their own day. It's easy to look back and ask: "Why didn't everyone adopt that sooner? What made people hesitate?"

I think one thing that makes people hesitate is a lack of access to expert information. Thus, part of my project with this book is to remedy that. Technology changes everything. We're said to live in the "information age" because it's easier to locate and access cutting-edge data than ever before. When it comes to important things—and certainly to our health—we need good, reliable information. Again, I want this book to be something that helps with that. I want to dispel the (few) inaccurate and exaggerated claims about CBD, and I want to reinforce the (many) true claims and breakthroughs that we are seeing every day.

I want to give you the tools to make definitive decisions, and not to hesitate. I want to assure you that the water is warm and safe and advise you to wade in with us. We are on the crest of a wave taking us to a future of greatly improved health and well-being, and I don't want you to hesitate. I don't want you—several years from now—to ask yourself: "Why the heck didn't I try that sooner? Why didn't I advise my loved ones to try that sooner? What was I afraid of?"

CBD is an industry that, in just the next decade or two, is going to revolutionize nutrition, healthcare, self-care, and more. From my position at the leading edge of the industry, it's challenging to give you "the view from here." "Here" is always changing. Things will have changed just in the time between my writing these words and when you read them. Tremendous infrastructures related to CBD production and distribution are being laid down. Laws are being written and rewritten to allow scientists to investigate the healing properties of CBD, and to allow consumers to decide for themselves if CBD is the right choice for them.

I think we're going to see something akin to the development of the telephone, the radio, or television in the next few years. That is to say, CBD will transform from something that might seem "new" or "strange" to the general population into something that most people have in their homes.

In my introduction, I said that we were in the early stages of a revolution. I hope that I've made my case for that. I hope you can see why revolutionary changes are going to happen— why they *have to* happen—considering what has been revealed about the awesome power of CBD.

CBD FAQ

I wanted to provide one more section here at the end of this book: a quick-reference FAQ that addresses questions about CBD that I may not have answered. Hopefully, this can fill in any blanks that may remain. (If you have additional questions that you don't see answered here, I encourage you to reach out to a qualified CBD authority.)

WHAT IF I ALSO LIKE THC?

It's a fact that many Americans enjoy using cannabis for the THC effect and are increasingly able to do so legally in the United States. And consumers who regularly use THC can also enjoy CBD when they wish to enjoy some of the benefits of cannabis without the intoxicating effects. When you combine THC with CBD from another source, it's important to monitor yourself for any changes as you adjust. If you are curious to learn more about the specific sensations to anticipate, talking to trusted employees at your local dispensary or marijuana store can be a good practical first step. Remember, like all substances we put into our bodies, drugs and medicines act, and interact, differently from person to person. Finding your own balance that keeps you feeling good and in good health may involve asking questions and a little trial and error. And when you find out what works for you, you don't have to keep it to yourself. Consider being a resource for others in your community as we all learn together.

Because of a growing interest in using CBD and THC together, legal growers have developed strains of smoking cannabis that have specially calibrated ratios of CBD to THC. The most famous among these is probably a strain called Charlotte's Web, which is famously low in THC, having a ratio of just 24:1 CBD:THC. If you are interested in adding THC to your CBD very gradually, a product like Charlotte's Web can be a great way to start small. As your body adjusts to the THC, you can move to other strains as you see fit. (Also note that the word "chemovar" is sometimes used by those in the know when discussing variants of cannabis and their CBD:THC ratio. If you see "chemovar," just think "strain.")

IF I TAKE CBD, WILL I TEST POSITIVE FOR A DRUG TEST FOR MARIJUANA?

No. If you use CBD obtained from a reputable source that has been manufactured correctly, you will not test positive for marijuana use. CBD contains entirely different components, and either no amount or only trace amounts of THC. There is still confusion from many people surrounding this question, however, because of other factors. One of these is the presence of cannabinol or CBN, another cannabis compound. Though far less prevalent, CBN is sometimes recommended for the same symptoms that CBD is suggested for, such as anxiety and sleeplessness. However, CBN is derived from THC and *will* create a positive drug test result for marijuana use. CBD and CBN are only separated by a single letter, and it's not surprising to me that people might confuse them. Another factor that leads to confusion, unfortunately, is intentional misrepresentation. For example, in the period we're currently living in, in which Americans are still learning about CBD, there are many misconceptions. Even those who know what CBD is are often far from experts. There are gray areas and sub-topics that still create great confusion. Because of this, there have been many high-profile cases of workers who have tested positive for marijuana use on drug tests yet insisted that the positive tests occurred because they were using CBD. I can tell you here and now, those people might have been using CBD, but they were not using *only* CBD. Again, there is essentially no way someone using CBD could fail a marijuana drug test. However, some people are happy to try to use public confusion to get a test result they don't like rendered null.

HOW MUCH CBD SHOULD I WORK UP TO? IS IT POSSIBLE TO TAKE TOO MUCH?

Researchers have experimented with giving test subjects both low and high doses of CBD to study very particular medical consequences, but the symptoms and doses studied are not exhaustive. As we reviewed earlier in this book, some people benefit from a targeted, relatively large dose of CBD to address a very specific situation. An example of this might be someone who does not regularly use high doses of CBD taking 150–300mg before engaging in public speaking or a similarly

stressful activity. However, most people who are looking to take CBD regularly will want to start with much lower doses. Anywhere from 5–30mg taken just once or twice a day falls into the widest category of use for those who take CBD as a supplement. Other than mild side effects, there is no general sense that taking "too much" CBD presents health hazards or is even possible to do. But to go back to our original follow-up question—Why are you taking CBD in the first place?—studies have shown that it is possible to lose beneficial health effects when too much CBD is taken. The best consumer is always an educated consumer, so I'd encourage you to investigate online resources and connect with people in a group or a community of folks who take CBD *for the same reasons you want to*. Their wisdom and knowledge can help you to make your own informed decision.

IF I HAVE MY OWN CANNABIS PLANTS, CAN I MAKE MY OWN CBD?

This is another case where I'm inclined to answer a question with a question. I have to ask: "*Why* do you want to make your own CBD from scratch?" I ask this because my initial inclination is to remind you that there are very sophisticated pharmaceutical-grade manufacturers who are in the business of making products that are very safe, with very specific dosing information, and delivering them to you in a safe, fast, and legal manner. But that much said, you may be a do-it-yourself-er.

You may prefer cooking a meal at home—even a very complicated one—to dining in a restaurant. If this is the case, I'm well aware that I'm not going to talk you out of it. But if you truly cannot be stopped, then I urge you to do your own research, learn what you are doing, and make safety a priority. Simply juicing cannabis leaves in your home juicer—for example—is not going to produce cannabis oil and is not going to do much in the way of releasing CBD. If you are genuinely interested in learning more about proper oil extraction methods, I strongly suggest you take the time to educate yourself on the resources available and begin saving up for the substantial financial investment it can take to purchase the equipment needed to extract CBD safely and effectively.

WHAT ARE MY OPTIONS IF I READ THIS BOOK AND I LIVE OUTSIDE OF THE UNITED STATES, OR IF I TRAVEL TO SUCH PLACES?

In this situation, you need to educate yourself about the options available where you live. In some nations, CBD, THC, and cannabis are legal to use for most people under most circumstances. Nations like the Netherlands and Israel, for example, have very enlightened attitudes about cannabis use. In other countries, they can carry direly serious legal consequences. The world is trending toward a greater acceptance and understanding of cannabinoids, especially CBD. However, you have to put your own safety first. Obviously, if you live outside of the United States, it's important to learn the rules and regulations of the country where you live. If you're traveling and wish to bring CBD with you, research the rules of the countries where you will be staying (or where you will have a layover).

WHAT IF I LIVE IN ONE OF THE FEW LOCATIONS WHERE CBD IS ILLEGAL, PRESCRIPTION-ONLY, OR OTHERWISE REGULATED WITHIN THE UNITED STATES?

First of all, take a deep breath, as this is a problem that can be solved. While CBD is now legal in most places in the United States, it's true that we have seen a few locations—cities, counties, or even states—that have shown they are still willing to push back against CBD in one form or another. The good news is that these laws have been largely ceremonial. What I mean by that is they do not genuinely prevent Americans from obtaining and using safe, nonnarcotic, nonaddictive, non-habit-forming CBD. Rather, they tend to be used so that politicians can make a point of showing that they stand with abstemiousness, regulation, and a pushback against modernity. If you live in a state where a law has passed requiring a prescription to purchase CBD, for example, you may indeed be prevented from purchasing CBD at the point of sale without one. However, nothing will prevent you from crossing state lines and purchasing CBD in a state where CBD is legal. Nothing will prevent friends or neighbors from bringing you CBD products when they come to visit. No law enforcement agency—local or national—has yet shown a willingness to crack down on consumers traveling to a different state to legally purchase their CBD. And between you and me, I think most people who work in law enforcement understand that there are "bigger fish to fry." Spending their limited time and resources to punish people for buying a dietary supplement and medicine that is legal in virtually every other place in the country is not a good move for any police department or law enforcement agency. If serious crimes spike at the expense of catching more CBD violators.[1]

I SOMETIMES SEE PACKAGING THAT ALLUDES TO DIFFERENT "TYPES" OF CBD. WHAT IS GOING ON HERE?

CBD is CBD. It is the molecule Cannabidiol. The differences revolve around how CBD is produced and extracted. As the consumer, you need to educate yourself and decide if these differences are meaningful for you or not. (Sometimes consumers find they can detect a great qualitative difference in these things. Other times . . . maybe they're just marketing.) One example is the difference between whole plant extracts and CBD isolate. CBD that

is extracted from whole plants is thought by many to be richer in healing compounds and liable to be more effective. CBD isolate is obtained from industrial hemp but believed by many to be less effective. Is there really a major discernible difference? Is it worth paying more for Whole Plant CBD extract? Again, some people have strong opinions in these areas, but for many consumers it will be a personal choice. Another area of similar ambiguity might be water-soluble CBD versus lipid-soluble CBD. Some people believe water-soluble CBD offers a more effective delivery experience for people who take CBD. Others find that they can detect no meaningful difference. I'm not here to tell someone they're wrong if they feel that water-soluble CBD has been a life-changing improvement over lipid-soluble CBD. However, I can say that the science and research needed to study and understand these differences has not yet been conducted.

WHAT DOES THE INDUSTRY LINGO MEAN WHEN IT SAYS SOMETHING IS "CBD-RICH" OR "CBD-DOMINANT?"

Throughout the marketplace, you are likely to see CBD and CBD-related products advertised as "CBD-rich" or "CBD-dominant." When used correctly, by honest vendors, these terms *should* have specific meanings. Namely, "CBD-rich" should indicate a cannabinoid product that has at least 4 percent CBD by dry weight. The term "CBD-dominant" should indicate that a cannabinoid product has a great deal

---

1 Please note that we are not recommending you break the law, but rather that there are other options available. However, always use caution and abide by the laws wherever you are living/staying/visiting.

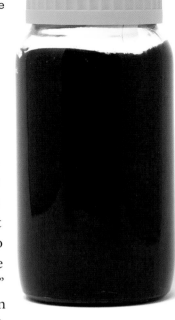

Whole Hemp Distillate

of CBD, but little or no THC. I say that these terms *should* correlate to the above meanings because the fact that CBD is so unregulated means that the terms are not currently legally defined or enforceable. For example, in the United States, food is heavily regulated by the FDA, so manufacturers must meet criteria in order to make certain claims. For example, for a food to be labeled "low sodium" in the US, it must have only 140mg of sodium (or less) per serving. For a food to feature the label "low cholesterol," it must have no more than 20mg of cholesterol per serving. However, because the FDA (or a similar entity) currently *does not regulate CBD products in this manner*, manufacturer claims are also unregulated. Does that mean you shouldn't trust the claims you see on packaging? Not necessarily. There's an old Russian saying: "Trust, but verify." I think that applies nicely here. When you're dealing with a new brand or manufacturer, or if a claim seems too good to be true, take the time to do some research before you take anyone's word about something. You'll be glad you did.

WHAT ABOUT THE TERMS "FULL SPECTRUM CBD" AND "BROAD SPECTRUM CBD"—WHAT DO THEY MEAN?

These are terms used by some manufacturers to indicate that the *entire* cannabinoid plant was used in the creation of the product you are buying. This would mean that the buds and leaves have been used, in addition to the stalks and stems. The research does not yet support the notion that supplements and medicines derived from certain parts of the plant are liable to be more effective, but many people seem to believe that this is the case. "Full Spectrum" can indicate that an entire plant containing THC was used, and "Broad Spectrum" can indicate that a plant containing no detectable THC was used.

CAN I DRINK SOCIALLY WHILE USING CBD?

The interactions of CBD and alcohol have been definitively studied. Generally, people taking regular doses of CBD are able to drink socially, within moderation, without issue. (Drinking to excess is a bad idea whether or not you are taking CBD.) If CBD and alcohol *do* interact, the anecdotal evidence points to the most common consequence being sleepiness. Many people take CBD for sleep issues, and some find that its effects can be rather immediate in this area. Because alcohol can also cause drowsiness, the effects of the two combined probably center in this area. Anyone having a drink for the first time after starting

CBD should be prepared for the possible side effect of feeling sleepier than usual. However, I will also note that some researchers believe that taking CBD could help to reduce the negative impacts of alcohol upon the body. For example, a 2013 study titled "Transdermal delivery of cannabidiol attenuates binge alcohol-induced neurodegeneration in a rodent model of an alcohol use disorder" found that CBD guarded against the cell damage normally caused by excessive alcohol consumption. In the study, lab rats given CBD in a gel form saw the damage to their brains from excessive alcohol decreased by 49 percent! Other studies have shown that CBD may protect against fatty liver disease, which can be caused by excessive alcohol use. (There have been studies that show cannabis—not pure CBD—can cause liver damage when taken to excess. It is important not to confuse the two here.) In addition, as noted earlier, there are studies that show that CBD can help people addicted to alcohol drink less or stop drinking entirely. At the end of the day, I think it's important to be informed about the relationship between CBD and alcohol. However, negative interactions between the two are not a major concern.

IS CBD VEGAN?

Yes, CBD itself is vegan. However, because CBD is often packaged in a gelatin-based delivery system, you should always check your product label if you maintain a vegan diet. Capsules and edibles are the two most common categories where nonvegan CBD shows up. Many capsules have an outer shell made from animal gelatin, and some CBD edible products—especially gummies—can contain animal gelatin. If you're vegan, the good news is that plenty of vegan capsules and edibles are also available.

I'VE HEARD THAT MY DOG CAN TAKE CBD . . . ?

You've heard right! Research shows that CBD can help dogs—and pets of all type—with a number of issues that can be frustrating for owners (and unpleasant for the pets themselves). The chemistry that reduces anxiety and inflammation in humans also seems to work for pets. Many pets can suffer from anxiety—either natural anxiety that's a hardwired part of their biorhythm, or incident-based anxiety from environmental sources like honking car horns or fireworks on the Fourth of July. Whatever the source, anxiety can make animals unfriendly and loud or make them act out in other ways (and even bring upon medical issues). Because unnecessary barking at noise can affect our neighbors in addition to our pets and ourselves, pet owners are looking for anything they can do to help their animals feel more relaxed. If you think your dog might benefit from CBD, talking to your vet can be a great place to start. Just keep in mind that— akin to physicians who treat humans—medical providers who serve dogs may, through

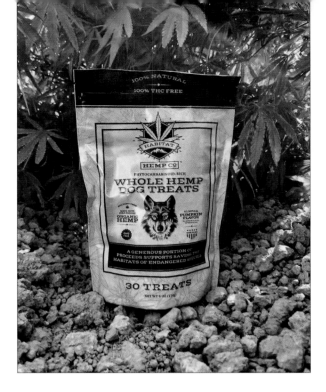

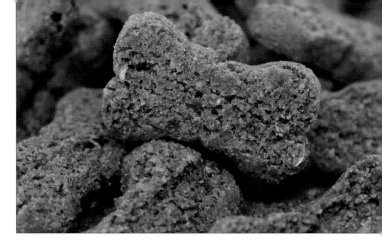

This up close shot of pumpkin, bacon, and full spectrum hemp dog treats showcases the quality of some of the snacks available for canines in need of the benefits CBD can offer.

no fault of their own, entertain ignorance and prejudice about CBD. Most state laws allow vets to discuss CBD for your dog if you bring it up. (Because of how some laws are written, your vet may hesitate to broach the topic if you don't do it first.) Only California has laws that explicitly *allow* vets to discuss CBD, THC, and/or cannabis as a possible treatment for pets. However, there seems to be more than anecdotal evidence that pet owners are hearing about CBD for dogs on their own. A 2019 survey by the Veterinary Information Network reported that nearly two-thirds of vets questioned said a patient had brought up CBD in the past month. To meet the growing demand for CBD for animals, manufacturers are responding with a wide variety of products specifically for dogs. CBD dog treats are popular and often come in flavors that dogs like, such as chicken, steak, and peanut butter. There is no agreed-upon "right amount" of CBD for pets, and many owners simply monitor

their dogs' response when working to get the dosage right. Despite this, many manufacturers will label their CBD products "for large dogs" or "for small dogs" and so forth. You will also find pet-focused tinctures that make it easy to place a few drops into your pet's favorite food. Is it possible to give a dog CBD products intended for humans? The short answer is yes, but buying dog-specific products may prove less of a headache in the long run. For example, getting a dose that is small enough can be an issue for pet owners. Even a dog that weighs 40 or 50 pounds—not a small dog by any means—will still require significantly less CBD than an average-sized human would to get a comparable effect.

What are the side effects for dogs? As with humans, side effects are typically rare and mild. Dogs might experience sleepiness or dry mouth manifested as increased thirst. (If these symptoms show up in your dog, try decreasing the dosage.) More research into the effects of CBD on dogs is currently underway. Earlier this year, the AKC Canine Health Foundation sponsored a study through the Colorado

State University's College of Veterinary Medicine and Biomedical Sciences on the effects of CBD on dogs. (Ironically, while previous tests of CBD have often involved animals, tests on dogs specifically have been relatively rare.)

Another important thing to keep in mind is that studies show dogs are very sensitive to THC. This is down to differences in the cerebellum and brain stem between dogs and humans. Dogs will be "hit harder" than humans by THC beyond mere differences in size and weight. Many pet owners who give their dogs too much THC have encountered a degree of toxicity that includes the dog being unable to stand or walk. Even vets who are well versed in cannabinoids for animals are cautious when using THC on dogs. All of which is to say, be very cautious if you want to treat your dog with a substance that contains

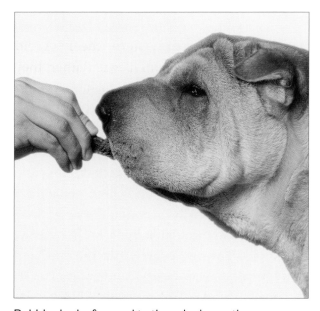

Buhbba looks forward to the relaxing anti-inflammatory benefits in his hemp treats.

both CBD and THC. Start with very small amounts of THC and watch your dog's reaction closely (while discussing thoroughly with your veterinarian).

WHAT IS KRATOM?

If you go to stores that sell CBD and CBD-adjacent products, you are likely to encounter kratom. Although some companies have made and marketed kratom infused with CBD, it is very important to understand that *kratom and CBD are not the same thing*. Moreover, if one is right for you, it doesn't necessarily follow that the other will be. Kratom is a dried, shredded leaf made from evergreen trees indigenous to Thailand, Indonesia, Malaysia, Myanmar, and Papua New Guinea. In indigenous cultures, kratom is chewed to relieve pain and increase energy. Kratom generally acts as a stimulant but is also known to produce opioid-like responses in some users. It can be taken in many ways but is most frequently eaten as powder (then washed down with a drink), consumed as tea, or eaten as a capsule. Proponents of kratom often cite its potential use as a painkiller for people with medical problems, and as an alternative to opioids. However, kratom remains very popular for recreational use. (Its popularity as a recreational substance began in Southeast Asia in the early 2000s and gradually spread to the United States and other countries.) The side effects of kratom are different from the side effects reported for CBD, which can include reduced appetite, insomnia, dizziness, and an increased heart rate. In the United States, kratom's status has always been more tenuous than that of CBD. In the opinion of many, it is a more serious substance with a greater likelihood of being abused. In 2016, the DEA reported that it intended to place kratom onto Schedule 1 of the Controlled Substances Act, which would have placed it in the same enforcement category as cocaine, heroin, and ecstasy. At the time, there was some disagreement over whether or not kratom deserved to be placed in the category. Eventually, the DEA backed down. However, the proposed Schedule 1 listing—and the ensuing controversy over it—encouraged many state and municipal politicians to take matters into their own hands. Consequently, several cities and states have made kratom illegal to buy or sell. In the meantime, kratom continued to grow its presence and often showed up in the same place that CBD was made available for sale. In 2017, the FDA took its turn attacking kratom, issuing a statement that no evidence supported its use as a legitimate treatment for opioid addiction and also noting that it had "significant safety concerns" about its use. Last year, the FDA issued even stronger warnings, saying that it now believed forty-four deaths had been linked to kratom and that kratom had no legitimate medical use. The FDA did not propose to ban kratom but—somewhat oddly—asked manufacturers to voluntarily withdraw from the US market. The FDA also prohibited the use of the term "safe" in connection with kratom by marketers, insisting that it has not been proved to be safe. Finally, this year, the FDA continued its aggressive stance with another warning, which read in part:

> FDA is concerned that kratom, which affects the same opioid brain receptors as morphine, appears to have properties that expose users to the risks of addiction, abuse, and dependence. There are no FDA-approved uses for kratom, and the agency has received concerning reports about the safety of kratom. FDA is actively evaluating all available scientific information on this issue and continues to warn consumers not to use any products labeled as containing the botanical substance kratom or its psychoactive compounds, mitragynine and 7-hydroxymitragynine. FDA encourages more research to better understand kratom's safety profile, including the use of kratom combined with other drugs.

Again, though certainly stern, the FDA did not move to make kratom illegal. Rather, they said that they felt it should not be used and would continue to warn people. (The FDA takes the same approach to tobacco cigarettes.) For the moment, kratom lies tangled in a regulatory web. Because of how it is used, it remains a substance that many regulatory bodies feel falls within their purview. Illegal in some states and major cities, kratom is also illegal to import, grow, manufacture, and sell in large quantities at different times and at different places. (Keeping ahead of kratom regulation is exceedingly challenging for anyone in the industry.) All branches of the United States Armed Forces forbid the use of kratom. It is very hard for anyone—even industry insiders—to confidently predict what regulatory agencies in the United States will decide to do next regarding kratom. With that said, if you live in certain states, you are going to see kratom sold and marketed as a CBD-adjacent product. I am not here to say that kratom isn't for you, but keep in mind that kratom is an entirely different substance from CBD, with its own entirely unique properties.

HOW DO WE KNOW CBD IS NOT ADDICTIVE?

CBD does not impact the parts of the brain that present any serious potential for addiction. It is possible that a person could become accustomed to CBD's positive effects and find that they are less physically sound and healthy when the CBD is taken away. However, strictly speaking, there is no potential for CBD addiction. (CBD removes pain, but not by getting someone high. If you have a pebble in your shoe, and you take the pebble out of your shoe, then your foot pain has been lessened or removed. Are you "addicted" to not having a pebble in your shoe? I would say no, you're not addicted; you simply find it preferable.) The 2017 study "Oral cannabidiol does not produce a signal for abuse liability in frequent marijuana smokers" settled the question of addiction for most people. Published in the *Journal of Drug and Alcohol Dependence*, this study tested the addiction potential of CBD by giving oral doses to people who regularly smoked cannabis. They found that CBD showed zero signs of being addictive, or even of hitting the same triggers for addiction as THC. (It is important to note that CBD alone is not addictive, but people who "get their CBD" by using cannabis that *does* contain high levels of THC may put themselves at risk for becoming addicted to cannabis.)

CAN MY CBD "EXPIRE" OR "GO BAD" IF I DON'T USE IT?

This depends on what form the CBD takes.

If your CBD product has container information about how long the product will remain potent—or an expiration date—you should obey it. Otherwise, it's a good idea to follow the same rules you would for most supplements or pharmaceuticals. Store your CBD products in a cool, dry place, preferably not in the direct sunlight. If your CBD products are in liquid form—such as a tincture—avoid a situation where light and heat might cause evaporation. If you use your CBD in capsule form, take care that the gelatin in your capsules does not break down.

CBD concentrate will not spoil and rot in the same way that food can. However, you always want to verify the physical integrity of the CBD you are taking. A capsule of CBD that is falling apart could lead you to take less than the recommended dose. A CBD tincture or liquid that is partially evaporated could have its CBD concentration affected, so you might be taking more (or less) CBD than expected when you use it.

My advice is to err on the side of caution. Given CBD's relative affordability, it just doesn't make sense to risk it with a product that may have compromised integrity. If you see signs like crumbling capsules, partial evaporation of a liquid, or hardening of a cream or salve, throw those products away and get something fresh.

THIS IS ALL INTRIGUING, BUT I "FEEL HEALTHY." SO WHY SHOULD I CONSIDER TAKING CBD?

Nobody should take CBD if they don't want to! It is clear that many people are able to live a full and healthy life without it. However, I would encourage you to consider the many prophylactic medications we take each day and ask yourself seriously how CBD has failed to establish itself as equally important to them. We take vitamins to help ensure we get all the nutrients we need, even if we haven't eaten a balanced diet that day. Men over forty often take a baby aspirin to help with heart and colon health. Because of the many positive things that CBD has been shown to do, I'd advise anyone to think about adding it to their daily supplements. We have seen how CBD helps with sleep. We have seen how it regulates anxiety. We have also seen how it boosts neurotransmitter function in the brain. In my opinion, you'd really be missing out if you never availed yourself of these benefits. Furthermore, even if the goal has nothing to do with healing or disease prevention, people who take CBD say that they just feel better. I'm not saying that hedonism is a good thing necessarily, but from a strictly hedonistic point of view, it makes sense to give CBD a try.

SOURCES
(*LISTED IN ORDER OF APPEARANCE*)

"VOTE HEMP RELEASES 2018 U.S. HEMP CROP REPORT DOCUMENTING INDUSTRIAL HEMP CULTIVATION AND STATE LEGISLATION IN THE U.S." [Vote Hemp press release]. January 28, 2019. Retrieved from: https://www.votehemp.com/press_releases/vote-hemp-releases-2018-u-s-hemp-crop-report-documenting-industrial-hemp-cultivation-and-state-legislation-in-the-u-s.

Gill, Lisa. "CBD Goes Mainstream." *Consumer Reports.* April 11, 2019.

Center for Behavioral Health Statistics and Quality. (2016). *2015 National Survey on Drug Use and Health.* Retrieved from: https://www.samhsa.gov/data/.

Center for Behavioral Health Statistics and Quality. (August 2019). *2019 National Survey on Drug Use and Health.* Retrieved from: https://www.samhsa.gov/data/.

Dahlhamer, James et al. "Prevalence of Chronic Pain and High-Impact Chronic Pain Among Adults—United States 2016." *Morbidity and Mortality Weekly Report.* September 14, 2019.

Opioid Overdose Crisis. [Webpage] January 2019. Retrieved from: https://www.drugabuse.gov/drugs-abuse/opioids/opioid-overdose-crisis

"RESEARCH WILL LEAD US TO A CURE" [CURE Epilepsy research webpage] Retrieved from: https://www.cureepilepsy.org/about-cure/mission/.

Mechoulam, R. et al. "Chronic administration of cannabidiol to healthy volunteers and epileptic patients." *Pharmacology* 1980; 21(3):175–85.

Koubeissi, Mohamad. "Anticonvulsant Effects of Cannabidiol in Dravet Syndrome." *Epilepsy Currents* 2017 Sep-Oct; 17(5): 281–282.

"FDA approves first drug comprised of an active ingredient derived from marijuana to treat rare, severe forms of epilepsy" [FDA press release] June 25, 2018. Retrieved from: https://www.fda.gov/news-events/press-announcements/fda-approves-first-drug-comprised-active-ingredient-derived-marijuana-treat-rare-severe-forms.

Norcutt, William et al. "Initial experiences with medicinal extracts of cannabis for chronic pain: Results from 34 'N of 1' studies," *Anaesthesia* Volume 59, Issue 5, May 2004: 440-452.

Corroon, Jamie and Phillips, Joy A. "A Cross-Sectional Study of Cannabidiol Users," *Cannabis and Cannabinoid Research* 2018; 3(1): 152–161.

M. Darkovska-Serafimovska et al. "Pharmacotherapeutic considerations for use of cannabinoids to relieve pain in patients with malignant diseases." *Journal of Pain Research* 2018 Apr 23;11: 837-842.

"NIH to investigate minor cannabinoids and terpenes for potential pain-relieving properties" [NIH press release] September 29, 2019. Retrieved from: https://www.nih.gov/news-events/news-releases/nih-investigate-minor-cannabinoids-terpenes-potential-pain-relieving-properties.

"Facts and Statistics" [ADAA website]. Retrieved from: https://adaa.org/about-adaa/press-room/facts-statistics.

"Generation Z." *Stress in America* [APA press release] October 2018. Retrieved from: https://www.apa.org/news/press/releases/stress/2018/stress-gen-z.pdf.

Ruscio, Ayelet et al. "Cross-sectional Comparison of the Epidemiology of DSM-5 Generalized Anxiety Disorder Across the Globe," *JAMA Psychiatry.* 2017; 74(5): 465–475.

Crippa, J.A. et al. "Neural basis of anxiolytic effects of cannabidiol (CBD) in generalized social anxiety disorder: a preliminary report." *Journal of Psychopharmacology* 2011 Jan;25(1): 121–30.

Blessing, Esther et al. "Cannabidiol as a Potential Treatment for Anxiety Disorders." *Neurotherapeutics* 2015 Oct; 12(4): 825–836.

Shannon, S. and Poila-Lehman, J. "Cannabidiol Oil for Pediatric Anxiety and Insomnia as Part of Posttraumatic Stress Disorder: A Case Report." *The Permanente Journal* 2016 Fall; 20(4): 16–005.

Linares, IM et al. "Cannabidiol presents an inverted U-shaped dose-response curve in a simulated public speaking test," *Brazilian Journal of Psychiatry* 2019 Jan–Feb; 41(1): 9–14.

"Mayo Clinic Q and A: Research needed into treating anxiety with CBD" [Blog Post] March 19, 2019. Retrieved from: https://newsnetwork.mayoclinic.org/discussion/mayo-clinic-q-and-a-research-needed-into-treating-anxiety-with-cbd/.

Olah, A. et al. "Cannabidiol exerts sebostatic and antiinflammatory effects on human sebocytes" *Journal of Clinical Investigation* 2014 Sept; 124(9): 3713–24.

Mounessa, Jessica et al. "The role of cannabinoids in dermatology" *Journal of the American Academy of Dermatology* July 2017, Volume 77, Issue 1, Pages 188–190.

Khanna, Raveena et al. "Cannabinoids for the treatment of refractory chronic pruritus." *Journal of the American Academy of Dermatology* October 2019, Volume 81, Issue 4, Supplement 1, Page AB29.

Murphy, Emily C. et al. "Knowledge, perceptions, and attitudes of cannabinoids in the dermatology community" *Journal of the American Academy of Dermatology* October 2019, Volume 81, Issue 4, Supplement 1, Page AB86.

"1 in 3 adults don't get enough sleep." [CDC press release] February 18, 2016. Retrieved from: https://www.cdc.gov/media/releases/2016/p0215-enough-sleep.html.

Carr, Teresa "The Problem with Sleeping Pills" *Consumer Reports* December 12, 2018.

Shannon, Scott et al. "Cannabidiol in Anxiety and Sleep: A Large Case Series" *The Permanente Journal* 2019 Jan 7. doi: 10.7812/TPP/18-041.

Babson, K.A. et al. "Cannabis, Cannabinoids, and Sleep: a Review of the Literature." *Current Psychiatry Reports* 2017 Apr; 19(4): 23.

Chagas, M.H. et al. "Cannabidiol can improve complex sleep-related behaviours associated with rapid eye movement sleep behaviour disorder in Parkinson's disease patients: a case series." *Journal of Clinical Pharmacy and Therapeutics* 2014 Oct; 39(5): 564–6.

Morgan, C.J. et al. "Cannabidiol reduces cigarette consumption in tobacco smokers: preliminary findings." *Addictive Behaviors* 2013 Sep; 38(9): 2433–6.

Hindocha, C. et al. "Cannabidiol reverses attentional bias to cigarette cues in a human experimental model of tobacco withdrawal." *Addiction* 2018 May 1.1

"Alcohol Facts and Statistics" [NIAAA webpage]. Retrieved from: https://www.niaaa.nih.gov/alcohol-facts-and-statistics

Prud'homme, Melissa, et al. "Cannabidiol as an Intervention for Addictive Behaviors: A Systematic Review of the Evidence," *Substance Abuse* May, 2015.

Gonzalez-Cuevas, G. et al. "Unique treatment potential of cannabidiol for the prevention of relapse to drug use: preclinical proof of principle," *Neuropsychopharmachology* 2018 Sep; 43(10): 2036–2045

Turna, J. et al. "Cannabidiol as a Novel Candidate Alcohol Use Disorder Pharmacotherapy: A Systematic Review" *Alcoholism: Clinical and Experimental Research* 2019 Apr; 43(4): 550–563.

Schubart, C.D. et al. "Cannabis with high cannabidiol content is associated with fewer psychotic experiences" *Schizophrenia Research* 2011 Aug;130(1-3): 216–21.

Zuardi, A.W. et al. "Antipsychotic effects of cannabidiol," *Journal of Clinical Psychiatry* 1995; 56: 485–486

Zuardi, A.W. et al. "A critical review of the antipsychotic effects of cannabidiol: 30 years of a translational investigation." *Current Pharmaceutical Design* 2012; 18(32): 5131–40.

Leweke, F.M. et al. "Cannabidiol enhances anandamide signaling and alleviates psychotic symptoms of schizophrenia" *Translational Psychiatry* 2012 Mar 20; 2:e94.

McGuire, P. et al. "Cannabidiol (CBD) as an Adjunctive Therapy in Schizophrenia: A Multicenter Randomized Controlled Trial," *American Journal of Psychiatry* 2018 Mar 1; 175(3): 225–231.

Boggs, D.L. et al. "The effects of cannabidiol (CBD) on cognition and symptoms in outpatients with chronic schizophrenia a randomized placebo controlled trial" *Psychopharmacology* 2018 Jul; 235(7): 1923–1932

Kogan, N.M. et al. "Cannabidiol, a Major Non-Psychotropic Cannabis Constituent Enhances Fracture Healing and Stimulates Lysyl Hydroxylase Activity in

Osteoblasts," *Journal of Bone and Mineral Research* 2015 Oct;30(10): 1905–13.

Nguyen, B.M. et al. "Effect of marijuana use on outcomes in traumatic brain injury," *The American Surgeon* 2014 Oct; 80(10): 979–83.

Russo, Ethan. "Cannabinoids in the management of difficult to treat pain," *Therapeutics and Clinical Risk Management* 2008 Feb; 4(1): 245–259.

Greco, Rosaria et al. "Activation of CB2 receptors as a potential therapeutic target for migraine: evaluation in an animal model" *Journal of Headache Pain* 2014; 15(1): 14.

"Cannabinoids suitable for migraine prevention" [EAN press release] *European Academy of Neurology* June 24, 2017. Retrieved from: https://www.ean.org/amsterdam2017/fileadmin/user_upload/E-EAN_2017_-_Cannabinoids_in_migraine_-_FINAL.pdf

Gong, H. et al. "Acute and subacute bronchial effects of oral cannabinoids." *Clinical Pharmacology & Therapeutics* 1984 Jan;35(1): 26–32.

Calignano, A. et al. "Bidirectional control of airway responsiveness by endogenous cannabinoids," *Nature* 2000 Nov 2;408(6808): 96–101.

Burstein, S. "Cannabidiol (CBD) and its analogs: a review of their effects on inflammation," *Bioorganic & Medicinal Chemistry* 2015 Apr 1;23(7): 1377–85.

Vuolo, F. et al. "Evaluation of Serum Cytokines Levels and the Role of Cannabidiol Treatment in Animal Model of Asthma," *Mediators of Inflammation* 2015;2015:538670.

Vuolo, F. et al. "Cannabidiol reduces airway inflammation and fibrosis in experimental allergic asthma," *European Journal of Pharmacology*. 2019 Jan 15;843: 251–259.

Calhoun, S.R. et al. "Abuse potential of dronabinol (Marinol)." *Journal of Psychoactive Drugs* 1998 Apr-Jun;30(2): 187–96.

Rock, E.M. et al. "Cannabidiol, a non-psychotropic component of cannabis, attenuates vomiting and nausea-like behaviour via indirect agonism of 5-HT(1A) somatodendritic autoreceptors in the dorsal raphe nucleus." *British Journal of Pharmacology* 2012 Apr; 165(8): 2620–34.

Bolognini, D. et al. "Cannabidiolic acid prevents vomiting in Suncus murinus and nausea-induced behaviour in rats by enhancing 5-HT1A receptor activation." *British Journal of Pharmacology* 2013 Mar;168(6): 1456–70.

Parker, L.A. et al. "Effect of selective inhibition of monoacylglycerol lipase (MAGL) on acute nausea, anticipatory nausea, and vomiting in rats and Suncus murinus." *Psychopharmacology* 2015 Feb;232(3): 583–93.

Rock, E.M. et al. "Cannabinoid Regulation of Acute and Anticipatory Nausea," *Cannabis and Cannabinoid Research* 2016 Apr 1.

Zamberletti, E. et al. "The Endocannabinoid System and Autism Spectrum Disorders: Insights from Animal Models," *International Journal of Molecular Sciences* 2017 Sep 7; 18(9).

Habib, Syed et al. "Role of Endocannabinoids on Neuroinflammation in Autism Spectrum Disorder Prevention." *Journal of Clinical Diagnostic Research* 2017 Jun 1.

Pretzsch, Charlotte et al. "Effects of cannabidiol on brain excitation and inhibition systems; a randomised placebo-controlled single dose trial during magnetic resonance spectroscopy in adults with and without autism spectrum disorder." *Neuropsychopharmacology* 44, pages 1398–1405 (2019).

Barchel, D. et al. "Oral Cannabidiol Use in Children With Autism Spectrum Disorder to Treat Related Symptoms and Co-morbidities." *Frontiers in Pharmacology* 2019 Jan 9; 9: 1521.

"NIH study finds extreme obesity may shorten life expectancy up to 14 years" [NIH press release]. July 8, 2014. Retrieved from: https://www.nih.gov/news-events/news-releases/nih-study-finds-extreme-obesity-may-shorten-life-expectancy-14-years.

Y. Le Strat and Le Foll, B. "Obesity and cannabis use: results from 2 representative national surveys," *American Journal of Epidemiology* 2011 Oct 15; 174(8): 929–33

Koch, M. "Cannabinoid Receptor Signaling in Central Regulation of Feeding Behavior: A Mini-Review" *Frontiers in Neuroscience* 2017 May 24; 11: 293.

Ignatowska-Jankowska, B. et al. "Cannabidiol decreases body weight gain in rats: involvement of CB2 receptors," *Neuroscience Letters* 2011 Feb 18; 490(1): 82–4.

Farrimond, J.A. et al. "Cannabinol and cannabidiol exert opposing effects on rat feeding patterns," *Psychopharmacology* 2012 Sep; 223(1): 117–29.

Parray, H.A. and Yun, J.W. "Cannabidiol promotes browning in 3T3-L1 adipocytes," *Molecular and Cellular Biochemistry* 2016 May; 416(1-2):131-9.

Jadoon, K.A. et al. "A single dose of cannabidiol reduces blood pressure in healthy volunteers in a randomized crossover study" *JCI Insight* 2017 Jun 15; 2(12).

Rajesh, M. et al. "Cannabidiol attenuates cardiac dysfunction, oxidative stress, fibrosis, inflammatory and cell death signaling pathways in diabetic cardiomyopathy." *Journal of the American College of Cardiology* 2010 Dec 14; 56(25): 2115–25.

Iffland, K. and Grotenhermen, F. "An Update on Safety and Side Effects of Cannabidiol: A Review of Clinical Data and Relevant Animal Studies" *Cannabis and Cannabinoid Research* 2017 Jun 1; 2(1): 139–154.

Pretzsch, Charlotte et al. "Effects of cannabidiol on brain excitation and inhibition systems; a randomised placebo-controlled single dose trial during magnetic resonance spectroscopy in adults with and without autism spectrum disorder." *Neuropsychopharmacology* February 6, 2019.

Sidney, S. et al. "Marijuana use and mortality." *American Journal of Public Health* 1997 Apr; 87(4): 585–90.

Johnson, JR et al. "Multicenter, Double-Blind, Randomized, Placebo-Controlled, Parallel-Group Study of the Efficacy, Safety, and Tolerability of THC:CBD Extract and THC Extract in Patients with Intractable Cancer-Related Pain." *Journal of Pain and Symptom Management* 2010 Feb; 39(2): 167–79.

Johnson, J.R. et al. "An Open-Label Extension Study to Investigate the Long-Term Safety and Tolerability of THC/CBD Oromucosal Spray and Oromucosal THC Spray in Patients With Terminal Cancer-Related Pain Refractory to Strong Opioid Analgesics," *Journal of Pain Symptom Management* 2013 Aug; 46(2): 207–18.

Pokrywka, M. et al "Cannabinoids—a new weapon against cancer?" *Progress in hygiene and experimental medicine* 2016 Dec 29; 70(0): 1309–1320.

Kiskova, T. et al. "Future Aspects for Cannabinoids in Breast Cancer Therapy." *International Journal of Molecular Sciences* 2019 Apr 3; 20(7). pii: E1673.

Ben-Shabat, S. et al. "An entourage effect: inactive endogenous fatty acid glycerol esters enhance 2-arachidonoyl-glycerol cannabinoid activity, published in the European Journal of Pharmacology." *European Journal Pharmacology* 1998 Jul 17; 353(1): 23–31.

Russo, Ethan "Taming THC: potential cannabis synergy and phytocannabinoid-terpenoid entourage effects," *British Journal of Pharmacology* 2011 Aug; 163(7): 1344–1364.

Grof, CPL "Cannabis, from plant to pill." *British Journal of Clinical Pharmacology* 2018 Nov;84(11): 2463–2467.

Rosner, Abbie "Cannabis for Parkinson's and Alzheimer's Diseases—An Interview with Dr. Ethan Russo," *Forbes* Feb 26, 2019.

"Dr. Ethan Russo: CBD, the Entourage Effect, and the Microbiome" [Project CBD Online Interview] January 7, 2019, Retrieved from: https://www.projectcbd.org/science/dr-ethan-russo-cbd-entourage-effect-and-microbiome.

Aidan J. Hampson, Julius Axelrod, and Maurizio Grimaldi (inventors) [2003] US Patent Number US6630507B1. "Cannabinoids as antioxidants and neuroprotectants" Retrieved from: https://patents.google.com/patent/US6630507B1/en.

Volkow, N.D. et al. "Don't Worry, Be Happy: Endocannabinoids and Cannabis at the Intersection of Stress and Reward." *Annual Review of Pharmacology and Toxicology* 2017.

Hua, T. et al. "Crystal Structure of the Human Cannabinoid Receptor CB1." *Cell* 2016 Oct 20; 167(3): 750–762.e14.

Simpson, Rick. *Rick Simpson Oil: Nature's Answer for Cancer.* Simpson RamaDur LLC, Amazon Digital Services LLC, 2016.

Zetlin, Minda "Coke With Cannabis? It Could Happen Sooner Than You Think" *Inc.* September 18, 2018.

Liput, D.J. et al. "Transdermal delivery of cannabidiol attenuates binge alcohol-induced neurodegeneration in a rodent model of an alcohol use disorder." *Pharmacology, Biochemistry and Behavior* 2013 Oct; 111: 120–7.

"FDA and kratom" [FDA press release] June 25, 2018. Retrieved from: https://www.fda.gov/news-events/public-health-focus/fda-and-kratom.

Babalonis, S. et al. "Oral cannabidiol does not produce a signal for abuse liability in frequent marijuana smokers" *Drug and Alcohol Dependence* 2017 Mar 1; 172: 9–13. ❦

INDEX

bone fractures, 65–67

Boston, 8

brain, endocannabinoid system in, 3

"brain fog," 88

brain health, 87–89

brain stem, 66

broad-spectrum, 169

bronchodilation, 73

brown fat, 84–85

Bush, George W., 14

butane, 132

C

Caldwell, Samuel, 9

California, 9, 14–15

cancer, 49, 50, 71, 76, 78, 89–95

cannabidiolic acid (CBDA), 76–77, 140

cannabinoid receptors, 2

cannabis
    high from, 1, 3, 36
    legal status, 8–13
    potency of, 15–16
    in United States, 6–21

CannaKids, 115–116

capsules, 142–143

cardiovascular disease, 84, 85–87

carrier oil, 140

Carter, Jimmy, 13

CB1 receptor, 2, 3, 5, 30, 47, 108–109

CB2 receptor, 2, 3, 4, 30

CBD
    addiction to, 174
    broad-spectrum, 169
    -dominant, 168–169
    drinking with, 169–170
    endocannabinoid system and, 1–5
    full-spectrum, 169
    homemade, 166–167
    irrepressible power of, 156–158
    production of, 130–133
    -rich, 168–169
    rise in use of, 19–21
    shelf life of, 174–175
    THC vs., 1
    tolerance to, 38
    whole-plant, 168

CBDA. See cannabidiolic acid (CBDA)

CBD oil, 120, 123, 124, 140–142

CBG, 116

CBN, 116, 165–166

cerebellum, 66

cerebral cortex, 66

Certificate of Analysis, 127

Charlotte's Web (cannabis strain), 165

chemical extraction, 132

chemotherapy, 66

chemovar, 165

Chicago, 7–8

Chinese medicine, 6

Clinton, Bill, 13–14

cluster headaches, 72–73